Oculoplastic and Reconstructive Surgery

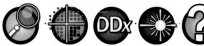

Rapid Diagnosis in Ophthalmology
Series Editors: Jay S. Duker MD, Marian S. Macsai MD
Associate Editor: Gary S. Schwartz MD

Anterior Segment
Bruno Machado Fontes, Marian S. Macsai
ISBN 978-0-323-04406-6

Lens and Glaucoma
Joel S. Schuman, Viki Christopoulos, Deepinder K. Dhaliwal,
Malik Y. Kahook, Robert J. Noecker
ISBN 978-0-323-04443-1

Neuro-ophthalmology
Jonathan D. Trobe
ISBN 978-0-323-04456-1

Oculoplastic and Reconstructive Surgery
Jeffrey A. Nerad, Keith D. Carter, Mark Alford
ISBN 978-0-323-05386-0

Pediatric Ophthalmology and Strabismus
Mitchell B. Strominger
ISBN 978-0-323-05168-2

Retina
Adam H. Rogers, Jay S. Duker
ISBN 978-0-323-04959-7

Commissioning Editors: Russell Gabbedy, Belinda Kuhn
Development Editor: Martin Mellor Publishing Services Ltd
Project Manager: Rory MacDonald
Design Manager: Stewart Larking
Illustration Managers: Bruce Hogarth, Merlyn Harvey
Illustrator: Jennifer Rose
Marketing Manager(s) (UK/USA): John Canelon/Lisa Damico

Series Editors: Jay S. **Duker** MD, Marian S. **Macsai** MD

Associate Editor: Gary S. **Schwartz** MD

Rapid Diagnosis in Ophthalmology
Oculoplastic and Reconstructive Surgery

Authors
Jeffrey A. Nerad MD,
Professor of Ophthalmology and Otolaryngology; Director, Oculoplastic, Orbital
and Oncology Service, Department of Ophthalmology, University of Iowa Hospitals
and Clinics, Iowa City, IA, USA

Keith D. Carter MD,
Professor of Ophthalmology and Otolaryngology; Chair, Department of
Ophthalmology and Visual Sciences, Oculoplastic, Orbital and Oncology Service,
University of Iowa Hospitals and Clinics, Iowa City, IA, USA

Mark Alford MD,
Oculoplastic Surgeon, North Texas Ophthalmic Plastic Surgery, Fort Worth, TX,
USA

Series Editors
Jay S. Duker MD,
Director, New England Eye Center, Vitreoretinal Diseases and Surgery Service;
Professor and Chair of Ophthalmology, Tufts University School of Medicine,
Boston, MA, USA

Marian S. Macsai MD,
Chief, Division of Ophthalmology, Evanston Northwestern Healthcare; Professor
and Vice-Chair, Department of Ophthalmology, Feinberg School of Medicine,
Northwestern University, Chicago, IL, USA

Associate Editor
Gary S. Schwartz MD,
Adjunct Associate Professor, Department of Ophthalmology, University of
Minnesota, Minneapolis, MN, USA

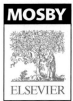

MOSBY

ELSEVIER

Mosby is an affiliate of Elsevier Inc.

First published 2008

ISBN 978-0-323-05386-0

British Library Cataloguing in Publication Data
A catalogue record for this book is available from the British Library

Library of Congress Cataloging in Publication Data
A catalog record for this book is available from the Library of Congress

Notice
Medical knowledge is constantly changing. Standard safety precautions must be followed, but as new research and clinical experience broaden our knowledge, changes in treatment and drug therapy may become necessary or appropriate. Readers are advised to check the most current product information provided by the manufacturer of each drug to be administered to verify the recommended dose, the method and duration of administration, and contraindications. It is the responsibility of the practitioner, relying on experience and knowledge of the patient, to determine dosages and the best treatment for each individual patient. Neither the Publisher nor the authors assume any liability for any injury and/or damage to persons or property arising from this publication.

The Publisher

your source for books,
journals and multimedia
in the health sciences
www.elsevierhealth.com

Working together to grow
libraries in developing countries
www.elsevier.com | www.bookaid.org | www.sabre.org
ELSEVIER   BOOK AID International   Sabre Foundation

The
publisher's
policy is to use
**paper manufactured
from sustainable forests**

Printed in China
Last digit is the print number: 9 8 7 6 5 4 3 2 1

Contents

Contents

Given the complexity and quantity of clinical knowledge required to correctly identify and treat ocular disease, a quick reference text with high quality color images represents an invaluable resource to the busy clinician. Despite the availability of extensive resources online to clinicians, accessing these resources can be time consuming and often requires filtering through unnecessary information. In the exam room, facing a patient with an unfamiliar presentation or complicated medical problem, this series will be an invaluable resource.

This handy pocket sized reference series puts the knowledge of world-renowned experts at your fingertips. The standardized format provides the key element of each disease entity as your first encounter. The additional information on the clinical presentation, ancillary testing, differential diagnosis and treatment, including the prognosis, allows the clinician to instantly diagnose and treat the most common diseases seen in a busy practice. Inclusion of classical clinical color photos provides additional assurance in securing an accurate diagnosis and initiating management.

Regardless of the area of the world in which the clinician practices, these handy references guides will provide the necessary resources to both diagnose and treat a wide variety of ophthalmic diseases in all ophthalmologic specialties. The clinician who does not have easy access to sub-specialists in Anterior Segment, Glaucoma, Pediatric Ophthalmology, Strabismus, Neuro-ophthalmology, Retina, Oculoplastic and Reconstructive Surgery, and Uveitis will find these texts provide an excellent substitute. World-wide recognized experts equip the clinician with the elements needed to accurately diagnose treat and manage these complicated diseases, with confidence aided by the excellent color photos and knowledge of the prognosis.

The field of knowledge continues to expand for both the clinician in training and in practice. As a result we find it a challenge to stay up to date in the diagnosis and management of every disease entity that we face in a busy clinical practice. This series is written by an international group of experts who provide a clear, structured format with excellent photos.

It is our hope that with the aid of these six volumes, the clinician will be better equipped to diagnose and treat the diseases that affect their patients, and improve their lives.

Marian S. Macsai and Jay S. Duker

Thank you for reading our book, *Rapid Diagnosis in Ophthalmology—Oculoplastic and Reconstructive Surgery*. We hope that this quick reference book will help you in your practice every day. If you are a clinician interested in common eyelid, lacrimal and orbital problems this book is for you. We have written the text with our background as oculoplastic surgeons, but the book is intended to be a "go to" source for dermatologists, otolarnygologists, plastic surgeons and family doctors, as well as ophthalmologists. Resident physicians and new practitioners should find the topics particularly helpful, pertinent and at an appropriate level. The text material can be used as a companion to other residency curricula and as a study guide for credentialing exams.

The topics have been chosen because they are seen frequently in the general population (like dermatochalasis) or because they should not be missed (like rhabdomyosarcoma). The chapters are short and intended to give you both the basic and the essential features of each topic without too much extra information. Each chapter begins with a key facts section that defines the problem, discusses the etiology and summarizes the important facts. At first read, you might get enough of what you need in these few lines, but if you need more, read on. Each chapter then details specific clinical features, diagnostic clues and ends with suggested treatment and prognosis. At the end of each chapter you should be confident of your diagnosis and know the direction of your treatment plan.

Conditions that affect the eyelids, lacrimal system and orbits are highly varied. Some conditions are life or vision threatening. Some are more of an annoyance to the patient. Some problems have a straightforward sight recognition diagnosis and a basic surgical solution (the lateral tarsal strip for an involutional ectropion lower eyelid), while complex orbital problems or cosmetic procedures demand patient input and depend on the surgeon's surgical experience and skill. Some chapters deal with the specifics of the surgical correction, but as a start we want you to focus on understanding the problem; the etiology, any anatomic or biologic abnormality, and the goals of treatment. In many cases you will have to move on to a more advanced surgical text to get the details for a specific procedure. No matter what the problem is, your skills of observation, diagnosis and treatment will grow throughout your career. We hope that this book plays a part in the learning process.

Jeff Nerad
Keith Carter
Mark Alford

We have many people to thank for their contributions to the production of this book. First and foremost, our thanks go to our families for putting up with the many hours away from home to keep up with our busy clinical practices. Many missed soccer games, volleyball games, piano concerts and dinners have been a part of our daily routines. Special thanks to Kristen and Elizabeth Nerad, Jodi Sobotka, Cheryl, Evan and Erin Carter, Ginger, Jake, Sam and Lee Alford. We love them all.

The education and clinical experience and required to write a book like this comes from many directions. The three of us all received all or part of our fellowship training at the University of Iowa. The granddaddy of Iowa Oculoplastic Surgery is Rick Anderson, so Rick is partly responsible for all of us. At least four more generations of "offspring" have followed from the Iowa program and all have contributed to the knowledge necessary to write this text. Although "the once a fellow, always a fellow" policy can always be invoked, one of the great parts of teaching is when a student becomes a colleague and a "teacher to the teacher". Others, have been very influential in our careers, too many to mention all, but including Richard Collins, John Wright, Dick Welham, Bob Kersten and Jack Rootman. At Iowa, we are fortunate to have a great faculty of colleagues to work and learn with. Our clinic staff make our lives easy seeing patients every workday: so many thanks to Teresa Espy, Sherry Brown, Deborah Kaefring, Pam Baye, Eileen Schmidt, Lacy Flores, Rosie Williams, Karen McDonald and Matt Hammons. The operating staff nurses have all contributed along the way too. Our daily interactions with our patients are what we really enjoy and without them, of course none of this would be possible.

Russell Gabbedy and Martin Mellor at Elsevier were great to work with. They had good ideas and did their best to keep us on schedule. Thanks to whole editorial staff as well, including the series editors, Jay Duker, Marian Mascai, and Gary Schwartz.

Lastly, thanks to all the many students, residents, fellows and colleagues that we have had the good fortune to share our passion for oculoplastic surgery with. We are looking forward to continue to learn from you in the years ahead.

Jeff Nerad
Keith Carter
Mark Alford

Acknowledgments

Section 1

Disorders of the Eyelid:
Congenital

Congenital Myogenic Ptosis

Key Facts

- Drooping of the upper eyelid(s) present at birth
- Several types of congenital ptosis—myogenic is most common
- Caused by dysgenesis of the levator muscle (Fig. 1.1)
- Unknown cause, rarely inherited
- Uncommon
- Occasionally associated with other ophthalmic or systemic abnormalities

Clinical Findings

- Variable amount of ptosis, ranging from mild (1 mm) to severe (4–5 mm or more)
- Unilateral or bilateral, often asymmetric
- **Clinical triad (Fig. 1.2):**
  - upper eyelid ptosis with weak skin crease
  - lid lag on down gaze (due to fibrotic levator)
  - reduced levator function (remember to stabilize brow when measuring)
- **Other clinical findings:**
  - may be associated with superior rectus weakness in a minority of cases; any other extraocular muscle involvement suggests a different diagnosis
  - not usually associated with any other extraocular facial abnormality

Ancillary Testing

- None

Differential Diagnosis

- Marcus Gunn jaw winking (elevation of ptotic eyelid with mouth movements due to fifth to third nerve synkinesis)
- **Blepharophimosis syndrome:**
  - congenital ptosis with blepharophimosis
  - epicanthus inversus
  - telecanthus
  - sometimes ectropion
- Congenital third nerve palsy (associated extraocular muscle paresis, may have aberrant regeneration)
- Congenital myasthenia (child with ptosis born to mother with myasthenia)

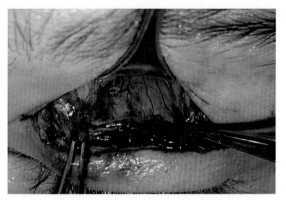

Fig. 1.1 Dysgenesis of the levator muscle, note rate fatty infiltration into muscle.

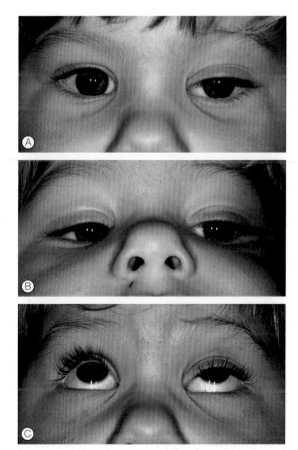

Fig. 1.2 Clinical triad (eyebrow should be stabilized at rim before measuring, not shown): (A) upper eyelid ptosis with weak skin crease, (B) lid lag on down gaze, (C) reduced levator function.

Treatment

- If not surgically treated, observe for amblyopia, especially if asymmetric
- If ptosis interferes with developing vision, perform eyelid elevation at earliest convenience, otherwise elective repair before starting school
- Surgical options (Fig. 1.3)
  - Moderate or better levator function (>4 mm): levator aponeurosis advancement
  - Poor levator function (0–4 mm): frontalis sling
  - Conjunctival Müller's muscle resection as an alternative for mild cases
- Lid lag and lagophthalmos are the rule after a sling procedure and may occur after significant advancement
- Corneal exposure is rare, even with frontalis sling, due to the excellent tear film and Bell's phenomenon in children

Prognosis

- Prognosis for good vision after surgical correction is excellent
  - Symmetry and cosmesis are very good, depending on amount of ptosis and presenting levator function (easier to fix with better levator function)
- Reoperation rate <10%, mostly indicated secondary to asymmetry
- In cases of moderate or poor function when an aponeurosis advancement has been performed, stretching of the muscle may occur, leading to recurrent ptosis

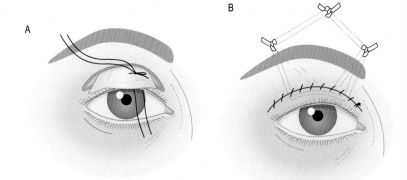

Fig. 1.3 (**a**) Treatment of ptosis with moderate or good levator function (>4 mm): levator aponeurosis advancement (note levator aponeurosis advanced over tarsal plate and sutured into place). (**b**) Treatment of ptosis with poor levator function (0–4 mm): frontalis sling, usually using fascia lata placed in typical double-triangle pattern.

Epiblepharon

Key Facts

- Congenital roll of eyelid skin pushing eyelashes toward the eye (*epi*, "on"; *blepharos*, "eyelid")
- Uncommon in general, most common in Asian eyelids
- Most cases do not require treatment
- Treatment is excision of the ellipse, of skin and muscle that pushes the lashes toward the eye

Clinical Findings

- Presents in early childhood with symptoms of eye rubbing or signs of irritation including conjunctival erythema
- In lower eyelid, eyelashes are pushed upward; in upper eyelid, eyelashes are pushed downward
  - The eyelid margin is in normal position
- More common in lower eyelid (Fig. 1.4)
- Eyelashes can be in contact with the cornea with the eyes in primary position or only on up or down gaze (Fig. 1.5)
- Punctate epithelial keratopathy can be present in area of eyelash touch
- Photophobia suggests significant corneal irritation
- **Other clinical findings:**
  - not associated with any other facial or systemic abnormality

Ancillary Testing

- None

Differential Diagnosis (Fig. 1.6)

- **Entropion:**
  - eyelashes turn against the eye
  - eyelid margin is turned inward also, either due to posterior lamellar scarring or involutional retractor and horizontal eyelid laxity
  - entropion rarely occurs in children
- **Distichiasis:**
  - an extra row of eyelashes emerges from the meibomian gland orifices, often turning upward toward the cornea (see *Distichiasis*)
- **Trichiasis:**
  - general term for any eyelid condition in which eyelashes are misdirected
  - often results from an unrecognized posterior lamellar contracture called marginal entropion (see *Trichiasis: marginal entropion and other causes*), in which subtle in-turning of the eyelid margin may be missed
  - misdirected lashes may also occur after trauma

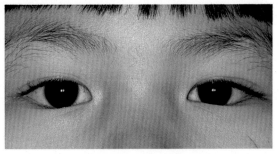

Fig. 1.4 Epiblepharon: a redundant roll of skin on the lower eyelid pushes the eyelashes toward the cornea.

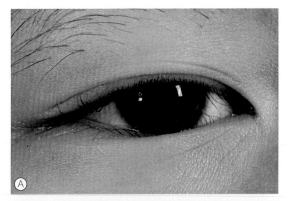

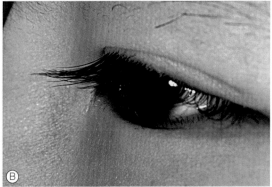

Fig. 1.5 (A) Front and (B) side views.

Treatment

- May resolve spontaneously as facial development progresses
- Topical lubricants for mild symptoms
- Indications for surgical treatment include bothersome symptoms or significant epitheliopathy
- A narrow roll of redundant skin and muscle is excised
  - The redundant skin should be pinched upward and marked
  - The excision should blend in with any epicanthal fold
- Complications of the correction are uncommon
  - Too much excision can cause ectropion or eyelid retraction
  - Too little excision may not correct the epiblepharon completely

Prognosis

- Reoperation rare—once corrected, epiblepharon does not recur

Fig. 1.6 Differential diagnosis of misdirected eyelashes. (**A**) Normal eyelid. (**B**) Marginal entropion (mild cicatricial): posterior lamellar scarring pulls margin in. (**C**) Epiblepharon: redundant roll pushes eyelashes against cornea. (**D**) Misdirected eyelashes: randomly oriented eyelashes aiming toward eye. (**E**) Involutional entropion: eyelid retractor and horizontal laxity allow margin to turn inward. (**F**) Distichiasis: two rows of eyelashes. (From Nerad JA 2001 Oculoplastic Surgery: the Requisites in Ophthalmology. Mosby, St. Louis.)

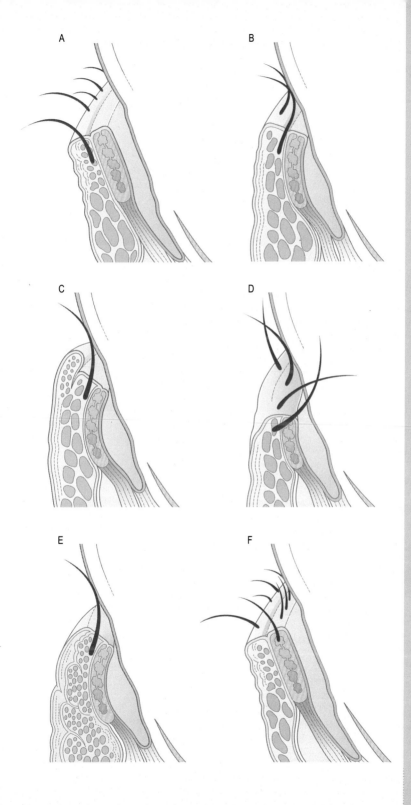

Blepharophimosis Syndrome

Key Facts

- **Narrowing of the eyelid fissures (blepharophimosis), occurring most commonly as a congenital syndrome of:**
  - blepharophimosis
  - ptosis
  - telecanthus
  - epicanthus inversus
- Unknown cause, autosomal dominant inheritance common
- Incidence uncommon, but one of the most common periocular genetic disorders
- Other facial and systemic abnormalities may occur
- Surgical correction of abnormalities, including telecanthus repair and ptosis repair (usually frontalis sling), typically performed around age 5 years
  - Lateral canthoplasty and lower eyelid skin grafting often necessary
  - If amblyopia is present, repair ptosis as soon as possible

Clinical Findings

- Blepharophimosis refers to horizontal narrowing of eyelid fissure
- Telecanthus is present without bony orbital abnormalities
- Upper eyelid ptosis is usually severe, with poor levator function
  - Ptosis associated with this syndrome represents a very small percentage of congenital ptosis cases
- Epicanthus inversus is a fold of skin that occurs over the medial canthus, extending from the lower eyelid to the upper eyelid
- Other clinical findings include ectropion of lateral lower eyelid
  - So-called lop ears (generous ears with helix overhanging slightly) can be found

Ancillary Testing

- Genetic testing for FOXL2 transcription mutation

Differential Diagnosis

- No other type of congenital ptosis is associated with these findings
- The findings of blepharophimosis syndrome may occur alone or in association with other genetic syndromes

Treatment

- Medical treatment rarely indicated
  - Amblyopia is rare because the ptosis is usually symmetric
  - Exposure from the ectropion rarely develops
- Begin correction of periocular abnormalities before school age
- Telecanthus repair usually performed with a transnasal wire
- Epicanthus repair should usually accompany the telecanthus repair
  - A number of procedures, including the "frogman" transposition flap technique (Fig. 1.7B) or the more simple Y to V procedures have been advocated
- Ptosis correction usually requires a frontalis sling procedure, usually done after any telecanthus correction
- Some cases may be treated with levator advancement if levator function is more than 4–6 mm (fig. 1.7B)

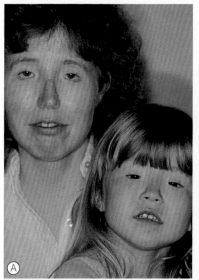
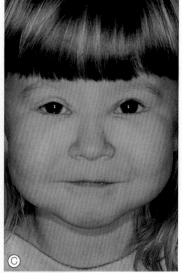
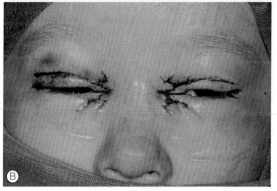

Fig. 1.7 (**A**) Mother and daughter with autosomal dominant blepharophimosis. (**B**) Intraoperative view showing eyelid crease incision for leavtor advancement and "frogman" canthoplasty. (**C**) Postoperative view. Note improvement of telecanthus but presence of scarring of canthi.

Blepharophimosis Syndrome (Continued)

- Lateral canthoplasty procedures are used to extend the lateral canthus beyond the orbital rim
- Skin grafting or lower eyelid tightening is used to correct the lower eyelid ectropion
  - Any combination of procedures is used depending on the individual patient
- Complications of lid lag and lagophthalmos can occur, as with any type of sling procedure
  - Corneal exposure is not common in children

Prognosis

- Sling operations generally successful in placing the eyelid in a functional position
- Cosmesis is improved but telecanthus and ptosis are usually not fully correctable
- Genetic counseling should be provided before childbearing age

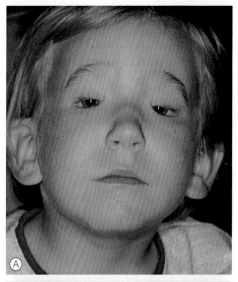

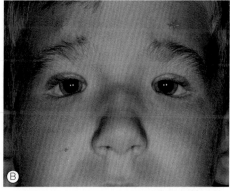

Fig. 1.8 Blaepharophimosis Syndrome. (**A**) Characteristic features of ptosis, epicanthus inversus, and telecanthus. Note elevated eyebrows and "chin up" position. "Lop" ears are present. (**B**) Postoperative view after sling procedure. Note improvement in MRD and deepened skin crease. Epicanthus and telecanthus have not been treated.

Distichiasis

Key Facts

- An extra row of eyelashes emerging from the meibomian gland orifices (*di*, "two"; *stichos*, "rows") • Caused by abnormal formation of eyelash portion of the meibomian pilosebaceous apparatus • Congenital, autosomal dominant, rare • If the patient is symptomatic, can be treated with cryotherapy, preserving the normal lashes using an eyelid-splitting procedure

Clinical Findings

- One or more abnormal eyelashes arising from the meibomian gland orifices, seen best on slit-lamp evaluation
  - Often several abnormal eyelashes are seen in one or more eyelid • A complete row of abnormal lashes is unusual (Fig. 1.9)
- The abnormal eyelashes may cause irritation from the corneal touch
- Generally not associated with other ophthalmic or systemic abnormalities, but there is a rare association with chronic lymphedema of the lower extremities

Ancillary Testing

- Genetic testing for FOXC2 mutation in lymphedema syndrome

Differential Diagnosis

- Can be confused with other forms of misdirected eyelashes, especially those conditions seen in children, such as epiblepharon (see Fig. 1.6) • Should be less confusion with entropion (eyelid margin turned inward) or other forms of acquired misdirected eyelashes (e.g. trauma) • Distichiasis sometimes confused with "dystichiasis" (suggesting misdirected eyelashes), a term that does not exist

Treatment

- If patient is symptomatic, surgery can be performed to destroy the abnormal eyelashes • Simple excision of eyelash roots from the posterior lamella can be used if only a few offending eyelashes are present • More commonly, eyelid is split into an anterior lamella (containing normal eyelash follicles) and a posterior lamella (containing abnormal eyelashes) • Cryotherapy is applied to tarsal plate to destroy the abnormal eyelashes (Fig. 1.10) • Some normal eyelashes are usually lost with the eyelid-splitting technique

Prognosis

- Excellent with lid splitting and cryotherapy

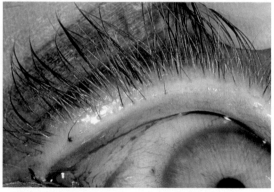

Fig. 1.9 Incomplete row of eyelashes emerging from the meibomian gland orifices.

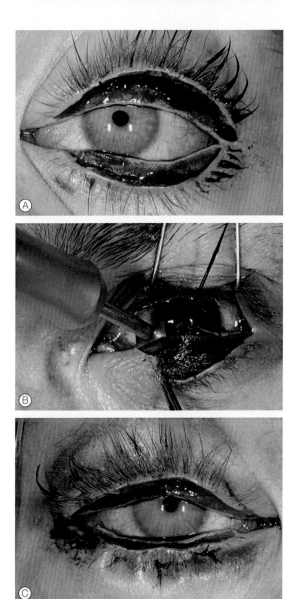

Fig. 1.10 Eyelid-splitting procedure (three different eyes shown). (**A**) Upper eyelid is split at the gray line. (**B**) Cryotherapy is applied to tarsal plate to destroy the abnormal eyelashes. (**C**) Anterior lamella is recessed. (From Nerad JA 2001 Oculoplastic Surgery: the Requisites in Ophthalmology. Mosby, St. Louis.)

Distichiasis

Eyelid Coloboma

Key Facts

- Congenital absence of eyelid tissue resulting from hypoplasia of embryologically adjacent tissues
- May occur as an isolated coloboma of the eyelid or as an extension of a facial cleft into the periorbital region (as classified by Tessier)
- Upper eyelid colobomas are often associated with Goldenhar syndrome
- Lateral lower eyelid colobomas most commonly seen in Treacher Collins syndrome
- Cause is unknown
- Colobomas are seen infrequently

Clinical Findings

- Upper eyelid colobomas are associated with corneal exposure
  - Defects range from very small to the entire eyelid (Fig. 1.11)
  - Edges of the coloboma may be adherent to the globe
- Lower eyelid colobomas associated with medial facial clefts can disrupt the canaliculus and nasolacrimal duct (Fig. 1.12)
- Goldenhar syndrome (oculoauriculovertebral dysplasia) is a developmental disorder of the first and second branchial arches (Fig. 1.13)
  - Typical facial features include upper eyelid coloboma, corneal dermoid, orbital lipodermoid, preauricular skin tags, auricular abnormalities, and mandibular aplasia or hypoplasia
  - Strabismus, nasolacrimal duct obstruction, and ptosis have been reported
  - Abnormalities commonly occur in vertebral column and auditory system
  - Palatal and facial clefts are common
  - Less commonly, the genitourinary and cardiopulmonary systems are affected
  - Most cases occur sporadically
- Treacher Collins syndrome (mandibulofacial dysostosis) is among the most common facial clefting disorders
  - Typical features include lateral lower eyelid coloboma, antimongoloid slant to eyelid, mandibular and zygomatic hypoplasia
  - A typical bird-like facies is present, partially due to a receding chin
  - Transmitted as an autosomal dominant trait linked to 5q31.1–q33.3

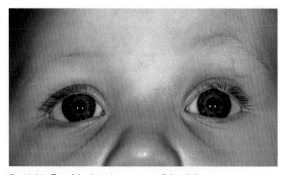

Fig. 1.11 Small isolated upper eyelid coloboma.

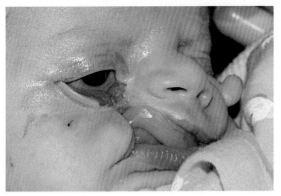

Fig. 1.12 Facial cleft associated with medial canthal dystopia, lower eyelid coloboma, and abnormalities of the nasolacrimal duct.

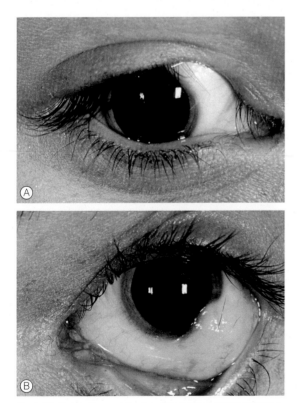

Fig. 1.13 Goldenhar syndrome: (A) upper eyelid coloboma, right upper eyelid and (B) corneal dermoid, left eye.

Eyelid Coloboma (Continued)

Ancillary Testing

- Systemic work-up if Goldenhar syndrome suspected
- Genetic evaluation for Treacher Collins syndrome
- Monitor for amblyopia

Differential Diagnosis

- Facial clefting disorders and various unusual facial syndromes may have associated eyelid coloboma

Treatment

- **Medical treatment of eyelid colobomas includes:**
  - lubrication
  - moisture chambers
  - monitoring for or treating amblyopia
- Surgical technique for repair depends on size and position of the coloboma
- Timing of the repair depends on presence and degree of corneal exposure
- Standard lid reconstructive procedures ranging from primary closure of the eyelid margin with cantholysis to entire reconstruction of the eyelid are used (Fig. 1.14)
  - Reconstructive options that do not include temporary occlusion of the visual axis are preferred

Prognosis

- Most colobomas seen by ophthalmologists are relatively small and easily repaired
  - If scarring of the cornea is avoided, amblyopia can be prevented
- Rarely, patient may have associated severe facial deformities

SECTION 1 • Disorders of the Eyelid: Congenital

18

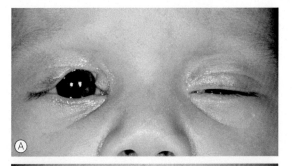

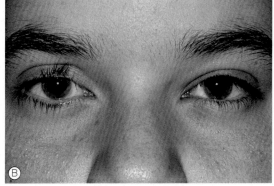

Fig. 1.14 Moderate size upper eyelid coloboma: (**A**) at birth, then repaired in the first few months of life; (**B**) 15 years later.

Section 2
Disorders of the Eyelid:
Lesions

Blepharitis

Key Facts

- **Summary:** inflammation of the eyelid margin
- **Pathogenesis:** most commonly caused by toxins and enzymes produced by *Staphylococcus aureus*, causing alterations in sebaceous secretions and resulting in poor tear film and inflammatory changes of the eyelid
- **Cause:** poorly understood
- **Frequency:** common
- **Other important considerations:**
  - frequently divided into staphylococcal and seborrheic blepharitis
  - patients with seborrheic blepharitis have seborrheic dermatitis (oily, erythematous, scaly scalp and skin lesions)
  - acne rosacea also a cause of blepharitis
- **Symptoms:**
  - itching
  - irritation
  - burning
  - tearing
  - blurred vision
  - red eyes
  - chalazion or stye formation

Clinical Findings

- Bilateral, seen in all age groups, more common in older adults
- Erythema, telangiectasias, and dilated vessels present along eyelid margin
- Thickened eyelid margins covered with oily yellow or white crusting or debris surrounding the lash base (collarettes), lash loss (madarosis) in more severe cases
- Abnormal sebaceous material may be expressed from dilated meibomian glands

Ancillary Testing

- Cultures and biopsies rarely indicated

Differential Diagnosis

- Facial rosacea
- **Viral infection (herpes simplex or zoster):** typically has skin ulcerations
- **Meibomian gland carcinomas**
  - consider in all unilateral cases
  - consider in any case that does not respond to treatment
- **Discoid lupus erythematosus:** lash loss and erythema

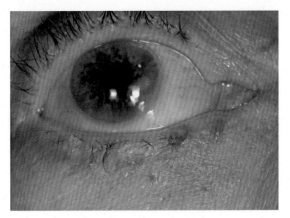

Fig. 2.1 Debris associated with seborrheic blepharitis along the right lower eyelid.

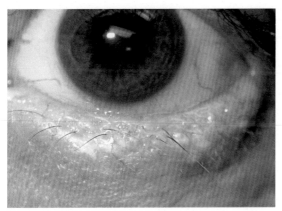

Fig. 2.2 A thickening of the lower eyelid as well as lash loss.

Blepharitis

Treatment

- Medical
  - Aggressive lid hygiene: warm wet compresses to eyelid margins followed by cleaning eyelashes and eyelid margins with a gentle dilute soap (e.g. baby shampoo)
  - Topical ophthalmic antibiotic: erythromycin or bacitracin to reduce number of bacteria; in more severe cases, antibiotic steroid preparation may be indicated to decrease inflammation as well (lifetime treatment may be required)
  - Systemic: oral doxycycline (100 mg p.o. b.i.d.) for more severe cases and those associated with acne rosacea; thought to stabilize meibomian gland secretions by inhibition of bacteria enzymes (lower doses, e.g. 20 mg b.i.d., may be used for maintenance)
  - Look for signs of facial rosacea and refer to dermatologist if suspected
- Surgical
  - Incision and drainage may be indicated if chalazia occur

Prognosis

- Good, but blepharitis is a chronic condition that is controlled, not cured
  - Intermittent flare-ups occur
  - Patients tend to do best if they follow a steady regimen independent of symptoms

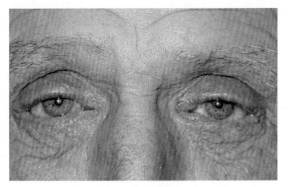

Fig. 2.3 Inflamed eyelids associated with blepharitis.

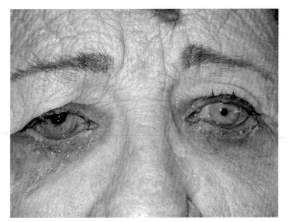

Fig. 2.4 Severe seborrheic blepharitis.

Chalazion and Hordeolum

Key Facts

- Localized inflammation and infection of sebaceous glands of eyelids
- **Pathogenesis:** obstruction of sebaceous glands (meibomian or Zeis) of the eyelid allows infection (hordeolum)
  - Sequestration of the inflammation may result in a non-tender, non-inflamed eyelid mass (chalazion)
- **Risk factors:**
  - blepharitis
  - acne rosacea
  - alterations in hormonal status (puberty, pregnancy, oral contraceptives)
- Extremely common
- Recurrent lesions or those that do not respond to appropriate treatment require biopsy to rule out sebaceous gland carcinoma

Clinical Findings

- **Hordeolum:** acute, suppurative inflammation producing a raised, erythematous, often tender nodule
  - Internal hordeolum: infection of the meibomian gland
  - External hordeolum: infection of the gland of Moll or Zeis
- **Chalazion:** firm, usually non-tender, localized nodule under the pretarsal skin
  - Often the result of an incompletely resolved hordeolum of a meibomian gland
  - Mass may extend through tarsus and be visible through the tarsal conjunctiva

Ancillary Testing

- Cultures rarely indicated
  - Biopsy required for recurrent or atypical lesions

Differential Diagnosis

- Neoplastic, inflammatory, and infectious lesions can mimic chalazion or hordeolum
  - Sebaceous, basal, or squamous cell carcinoma
  - Molluscum contagiosum, tuberculosis, sarcoidosis, epithelial inclusion cysts

Treatment

- Medical therapy
  - Limited efficacy
  - More beneficial at preventing future episodes in patients with recurrent disease
  - Eyelid hygiene: warm compresses directly to lesion to melt lipid secretions and reverse plugging; cleaning with dilute (one drop per 5 cc of water) baby shampoo to remove oily debris, decrease bacterial load, and control blepharitis
  - Topical ophthalmic antibiotic ointment is minimally effective—consider antibiotic–steroid combination
  - Oral antibiotic (doxycycline 100 mg p.o. b.i.d.) if acne rosacea present; if lesions occur over eyelids on a chronic basis, oral antibiotic treatment may be indicated indefinitely

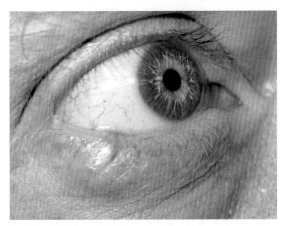

Fig. 2.5 Chalazion of right lower eyelid. Note absence of inflammation.

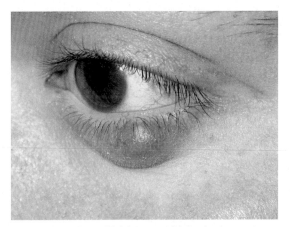

Fig. 2.6 Hordeolum of left lower eyelid. Lesion is erythematous and tender.

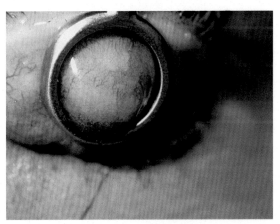

Fig. 2.7 Everted eyelid with chalazion clamp in place.

- Surgical
  - Drainage and curettage if medical therapy fails
  - Best performed via conjunctival surface with a chalazion clamp in place (Fig. 2.7): use a no. 11 blade to open chalazion with a vertical incision; scoop out contents with a curette (Fig. 2.8)
  - Intralesional injection of steroid can be effective
- **Complications:**
  - gland dropout
  - eyelash loss
  - eyelid margin changes
  - ptosis
  - conjunctival scar

Prognosis

- Most cases respond to medical and/or surgical treatment with no long-term complications
  - Patients with rosacea may have recurrent disease
- Recurrence rate high if underlying blepharitis or meibomianitis not treated with chronic eyelid hygiene (see above)

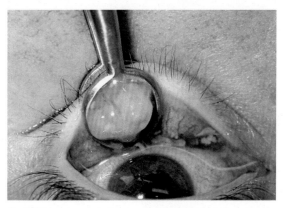

Fig. 2.8 Lipogranulomatous contents of a chalazion during excision.

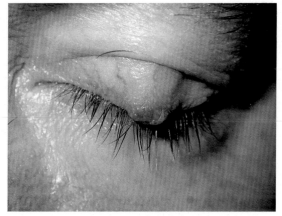

Fig. 2.9 Hordeolum at eyelid margin.

Seborrheic Keratosis

Key Facts
- Most common skin lesion, common in periocular area
- Benign neoplasm
- Middle-aged to older patients

Clinical Findings
- Lesions are brown to dark brown warty plaques
- Lesion has a greasy, stuck-on appearance, especially away from the thin eyelid skin (Fig. 2.10)
- Eyelid skin lesions tend to appear pedunculated or papillary rather than flat (Fig. 2.11)

Ancillary Testing
- None

Differential Diagnosis
- Malignant melanoma if darkly or asymmetrically pigmented
- Epidermal nevus
- Verruca vulgaris
- Acrochordon (skin tag)

Treatment
- Observation if sure of diagnosis
- Biopsy if lesion is symptomatic, catching clothing
- Shave biopsy works well
  - Cryotherapy can be effective

Prognosis
- Excellent, low recurrence rate

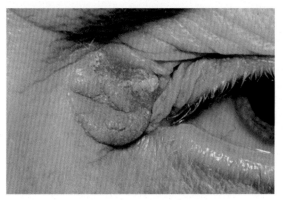

Fig. 2.10 Brown, warty-looking lesion with classic stuck-on appearance of seborrheic keratosis.

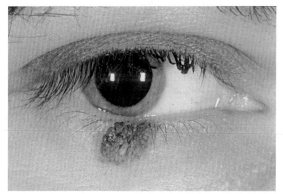

Fig. 2.11 Brownish black pedunculated papillary lesion of the right lower eyelid.

Epidermal Inclusion Cyst

Key Facts

- Occurs when epithelial cells are turned inward, buried within the skin
  - The epidermal wall sheds keratin
- Usually the result of entrapment of epithelial cells of the infundibulum of the hair follicle
  - May occur after trauma if the skin surface is interrupted
- Common benign lesion in periocular area

Clinical Findings

- Lesion appears smooth (Fig. 2.12), and a central pore may be present
- Slowly enlarges as the cyst wall produces keratin (not sebaceous material)
- Can be associated with minor skin trauma

Ancillary Testing

- None

Differential Diagnosis

- Neurofibroma

Treatment

- Observation
- Marsupialization of cyst is simple and effective
- If complete excision of cyst is attempted, the entire cyst wall must be removed to prevent recurrence

Prognosis

- Excellent with marsupialization or complete cyst excision

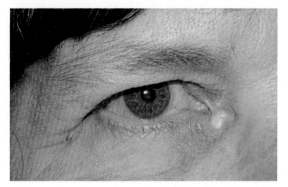

Fig. 2.12 Smooth, elevated, whitish lesion in the right medial canthus.

Xanthelasma

Key Facts

- Common skin lesion of the medial aspect of upper and lower eyelids
- Middle-aged to older patients
- Usually bilateral
- Usually not associated with hyperlipidemic condition

Clinical Findings

- Yellowish dermal plaques of the eyelids (Fig. 2.13)
- Lesion is composed of lipid-laden macrophages
- Upper lids more common location

Ancillary Testing

- Serum lipid levels if suspected metabolic disorder

Differential Diagnosis

- Usually no other lesions look like this, but some other xanthematous lesions may appear yellow

Treatment

- Full-thickness excision of lesion
- Must be careful not to remove too much of the anterior lamella of the eyelid
- Must avoid lagophthalmos and ectropion with skin closure
- Carbon dioxide laser ablation or trichloroacetic acid is less likely to be effective, because the lesion extends deep into the dermis
- Full-thickness skin grating may be required after excision of larger lesions

Prognosis

- Excellent with surgical excision
- Recurrence possible

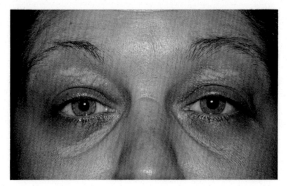

Fig. 2.13 A 49-year-old woman with yellowish plaques in all four eyelids.

Nevus

Key Facts

- Common lesion of the eyelid
- Appearance depends on skin level where nevus resides
- Nevus cells arise from undifferentiated melanocytes
- Nevi not normally present at birth
- Nevi usually appear and can increase in size and change in pigmentation during puberty
- Three stages of a nevus
  1. Junctional: at junction of epidermis and dermis
  2. Compound: in epidermis extending deeper into dermis
  3. Dermal: solely in dermis

Clinical Findings

- **Children:** nevi usually flat pigmented macules
  - This stage is junctional, usually appearing in adolescence
- **Middle-aged adults:** elevated lesion, pigmented lesion compound stage. The pigment is slowly lost as the nevus ages (Fig. 2.14)
- **Older patients:**
  - dermal stage
  - pigment usually lost
  - lesion appears elevated in a dome shape
- A common location is the eyelid margin
- Eyelid margin structures are not destroyed, as with carcinomas
  - Eyelashes grow out through the nevus but may lose their parallel orientation (Fig. 2.15)

Ancillary Testing

- None. See below for indications for biopsy

Differential Diagnosis

- Pigmented seborrheic keratosis
- Melanoma (see below)

Treatment

- Observation
- Simple shave biopsy removes any elevated portion (may mean slowly)
- Wedge resection of the eyelid margin or excisional biopsy at full thickness eyelid skin for complete removal

Prognosis

- Excellent
- If only superficial portion is removed, the nevus may recur over time
- **Biopsy recommended if melanoma suspected:**
  - large lesions (>6 mm)
  - bleeding
  - highly irregular borders
  - change in pigmentation

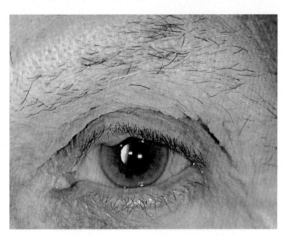

Fig. 2.14 Elevated nevus of the left upper eyelid in a middle-aged patient. Note no loss of eyelid margin architecture.

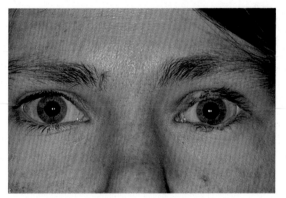

Fig. 2.15 Nevus of the left upper eyelid. Note lashes growing through the nevus and spreading individual lashes apart.

Actinic Keratosis

Key Facts

- Most common precancerous skin lesion
- Associated with chronic sun exposure
- More common in patients with light complexion

Clinical Findings

- Lesions are scaly hyperkeratotic plaques that may flake off and reappear
- Lesions can arise on any sun-exposed skin
- **Common locations:**
  - face • neck • forearms • ears • hands

Ancillary Testing

- Excisional biopsy

Differential Diagnosis

- Seborrheic keratosis
- Early squamous cell carcinoma appears hyperkeratotic

Treatment

- Simple excisional biopsy is a typical treatment in periocular area
- Treatment away from the periocular region usually consists of liquid nitrogen application
- Alternative treatments, especially for numerous lesions, include topical 5-flurouracil or chemical peeling
- Sunscreen recommended

Prognosis

- Excellent
- Low malignant potential
  - With proper treatment, risk of progression to squamous cell carcinoma is quite low
- Other actinic lesions (e.g. basal cell carcinoma or squamous cell carcinoma) should be screened for in these patients

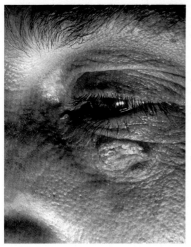

Fig. 2.16 Scaly plaque-like lesion on left lower eyelid.

Keratoacanthoma

Key Facts

- Rapidly developing lesion (weeks)
- Affects middle-aged to older patients
- Cause unknown, possibly trauma or sunlight exposure
- Historically was thought of as a benign lesion
- May represent low-grade squamous cell carcinoma

Clinical Findings

- Rapidly growing lesion with central crater filled with keratin and with rounded margins (Fig. 2.17)
- Usually located on lower eyelid (Fig. 2.18)
- Lesions said to spontaneously involute
  - Surgical removal usually performed before allowing involution

Ancillary Testing

- None

Differential Diagnosis

- Basal cell carcinoma
- Squamous cell carcinoma

Treatment

- Excision of lesion
- Send to pathology for definitive diagnosis

Prognosis

- Excellent—recurrences are rare

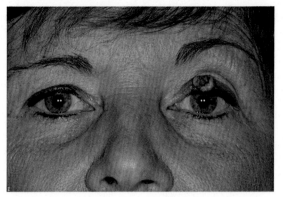

Fig. 2.17 More advanced lesion (compared with that in Fig. 2.18) on left upper eyelid, with more keratin filling the central crater.

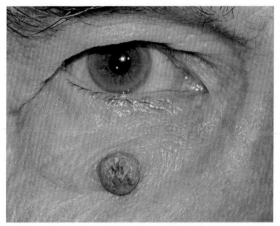

Fig. 2.18 Dome-shaped lesion with central crater on right lower eyelid.

Lentigo Maligna

Key Facts

- Also called Hutchinson melanotic freckle
- Lesion has varied pigmentation and irregular borders
- Progressive growth can lead to melanoma

Clinical Findings

- Presents as flat, pigmented lesion with irregular border (Fig. 2.19)
- Periocular area is common location
- Seen in older patients
- Can extend on to conjunctiva and appear as primary acquired melanosis
- Progressive growth with increasing pigmentation
- 30–50% of these lesion will progress to invasive melanoma
- **Malignant transformation should be suspected:**
  - when there are significant changes in pigmentation, borders, or thickness
  - if associated with bleeding (see *Cutaneous melanoma*)

Ancillary Testing

- None

Differential Diagnosis

- Solar lentigo
- Lentigo simplex
- Melanoma

Treatment

- Punch biopsy for diagnosis
- Excision of lesion with controlled tissue margins (Fig. 2.20)
- Monitor patient for recurrent lesion
- Sunscreen recommended

Prognosis

- Good
- May recur
- Fewer than half of these lesions progress to melanoma
- Melanoma arising from lentigo maligna is more difficult to treat, because of diffuse spread of malignant cells

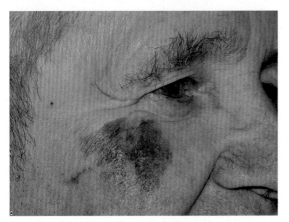

Fig. 2.19 Large lesion with various shades of pigment. Biopsies were consistent with lentigo maligna.

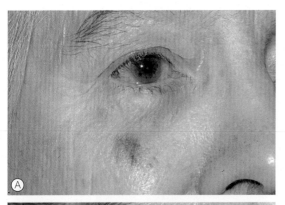

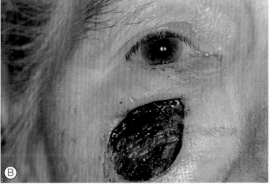

Fig. 2.20 (**A**) Pigmented lesion with flat irregular shape on the right cheek. (**B**) Surgical defect after lesion was removed with controlled margins. Microscopic margins usually extend well beyond clinical involvement.

Basal Cell Carcinoma

Key Facts

- Most common cutaneous malignancy
- Caused by ultraviolet radiation in susceptible persons
- Common in light-skinned populations
- Early diagnosis important
- Treatment by complete surgical excision

Clinical Findings

- Sun-exposed regions of lower eyelid and medial canthus are most common locations
- **Characteristic findings include (Fig. 2.21):**
  - irregular margins
  - rolled pearly margins (Fig. 2.21A)
  - central ulceration
  - telangiectasia
  - loss of eyelid margin architecture, including eyelash loss (Fig. 2.21B)
- Several subtypes exist
  - The nodular subtype is the most common (see Fig. 2.22A)

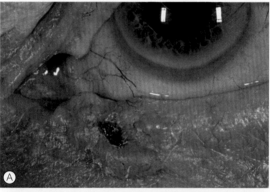

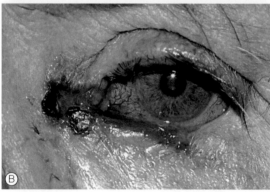

Fig. 2.21 (**A**) Typical nodular basal cell carcinoma with raised rolled pearly margins and central ulceration.
(**B**) More destructive basal cell carcinoma with loss of lid margin architecture.

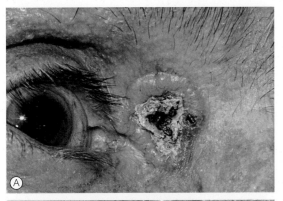

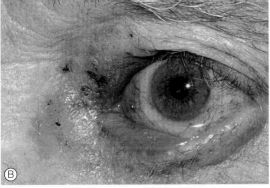

Fig. 2.22 (**A**) Nodular subtype: clinical margins are easy to see. (**B**) Morpheaform subtype, with non-distinct margins typically requiring a resection larger than predicted to clear the margins.

Basal Cell Carcinoma (Continued)

- Morpheaform, cystic, and pigmented subtypes also exist
  - The morpheaform subtype is the most aggressive and most difficult to diagnose (see Fig. 2.22B)
- Basal cell nevus syndrome (Gorlin syndrome) is a very rare autosomal dominantly inherited syndrome associated with multiple basal cell carcinomas
  - Dental cysts, skeletal abnormalities, palmar pits, and nail abnormalities may accompany

Ancillary Testing

- Incisional biopsy when malignancy suspected
- If signs of orbital extension suspected on clinical examination, CT or MRI is indicated

Differential Diagnosis

- Benign cutaneous lesions do not show the features of malignancy outlined above
- Other cutaneous malignancies, especially squamous cell carcinoma, can be confused with basal cell carcinoma
  - Characteristically, squamous cell carcinoma shows hyperkeratosis, whereas basal cell carcinoma does not
- If any uncertainty exists regarding whether a lesion is benign or malignant, an incisional biopsy should be performed (see Fig. 2.23)

Treatment

- Use of sunscreen and sunglasses and avoidance of sun exposure are helpful preventive measures, especially in childhood
- Excisional biopsy is the standard treatment
- Confirm free margins with frozen or permanent sections before reconstruction
- **Mohs surgery is a useful technique, especially for:**
  - morpheaform subtypes
  - canthal lesions
  - recurrent tumors
- Most reconstructions offer normal or near normal function and cosmesis
- Topical 5-fluorouracil or the immunostimulant, imiquimod (Aldara), may be useful for superficial tumors, especially when numerous lesions are present
- Radiation therapy can be used as a palliative adjunct in extensive or recurrent cases

Prognosis

- Surgical cure rate is >95%
  - Metastases do not occur
- Neglected tumors can grow to large size and extend into orbit
- Canthal lesions tend to have higher recurrent rate
- Patients should be observed for ≥5 years before a cure is recognized

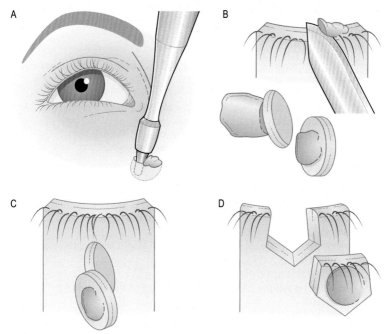

Fig. 2.23 Biopsy techniques. (**A**) Punch biopsy: a trephine is used in melanoma biopsy to assess the depth of the lesion. (**B**) Incisional biopsy: a portion of the tumor is sampled to confirm the clinical diagnosis. (**C**) Shave biopsy: a blade is used to shave off the elevated portion of a benign lesion—useful for seborrheic keratoses in the periocular area and nevi on the eyelid margin. (**D**) Excisional biopsy: all the lesion is removed and margins are evaluated; wedge resection of the eyelid margin is used to remove a malignancy on or near the eyelid margin. (From Nerad JA 2001 Oculoplastic Surgery: the Requisites in Ophthalmology. Mosby, St. Louis.)

Squamous Cell Carcinoma

Key Facts

- Malignant cutaneous neoplasm, less common but more aggressive than basal cell carcinoma
- <5% of periocular malignancies
- Like basal cell carcinoma, squamous cell carcinoma (SCC) is caused by ultraviolet radiation in susceptible persons
- Actinic keratosis is a premalignant form of SCC
- Potential for neurotrophic spread and regional metastases

Clinical Findings

- Lesions occurring in setting of sun-damaged skin should arouse suspicion of malignancy
- **SCC shows features similar to those of other malignancies (Figs 2.24 and 2.25):**
  - irregular margins • ulceration • loss of eyelid margin architecture including eyelash loss
- Hyperkeratosis typical (Figs 2.24–2.26)
- Rolled pearly margins and telangiectasias are not hallmarks, as in basal cell carcinoma
- Aggressive local growth pattern, often with indistinct margins that may necessitate a large resection
- Potential for perineural spread (Fig. 2.27)
  - Hypesthesia and formication are symptoms
  - Intraorbital or intracranial extension is possible
- Higher recurrence rate than basal cell carcinoma
- Check for regional node involvement at time of diagnosis and in follow-up

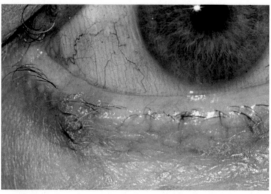

Fig. 2.24 Small SCC. Note hyperkeratosis.

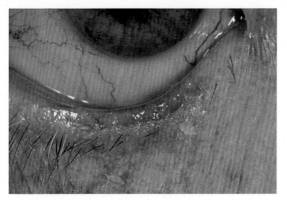
Fig. 2.25 Eyelid margin SCC with eyelash loss and ulceration.

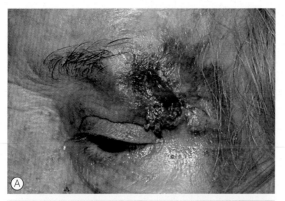

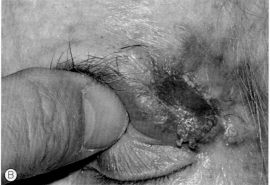
Fig. 2.26 Recurrent eyebrow SCC. (A) Note hyperkeratosis and area of healed ulceration. (B) Recurrent tumor was adherent to bone but did not extend through septum.

Ancillary Testing

- Incisional biopsy to make diagnosis
- Orbital imaging (CT or MRI) for suspected intraorbital extension or deep neurotrophic spread (Fig. 2.27B)
- Ear, nose, and throat consult for any suspected cervical node involvement

Differential Diagnosis

- Clinically, SCC may be confused with basal cell carcinoma
- Actinic keratosis may be difficult to differentiate from early cases of SCC

Treatment

- Use of sunscreen and sunglasses and avoidance of sun exposure are helpful preventive measures, especially in childhood
- Excisional biopsy with confirmation of free surgical margins is the standard treatment
- Reconstruction after confirmation of free margins
- Mohs surgery is a useful technique, especially for canthal lesions and recurrent tumors
- **Extensive reconstructions may leave some abnormality, such as:**
  - eyelid malposition or asymmetry • incomplete blink • scarring
- 5-Fluorouracil cream, the immunostimulant cream, imiquimod (Aldara), or photodynamic therapy can be used in patients with many premalignant lesions and early SCCs
- Cryotherapy can be used for actinic keratosis but is not a definitive treatment for SCC
- Radiation therapy is a useful palliative adjunct in extensive or recurrent cases but is not generally considered a primary treatment

Prognosis

- Cure rate is high but lower than that for basal cell carcinoma
- Neurotrophic spread is a limiting factor in curing patients
- Patients should be observed for ≥ 5 years before a cure is recognized

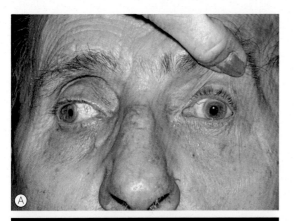

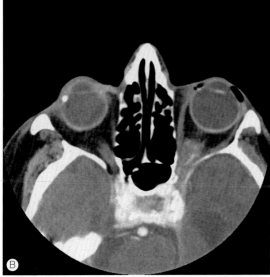

Fig. 2.27 Intracranial neurotrophic spread due to recurrent SCC originating on the temple. (**A**) Third nerve palsy due to orbital apex and cavernous sinus spread. (**B**) CT scan showing extension into orbital apex and cavernous sinus.

Sebaceous Adenocarcinoma

Key Facts

- Malignant neoplasm arising from a sebaceous gland, usually the meibomian gland
- Frequently called sebaceous cell carcinoma
- Misdiagnosed because of a variable appearance that may resemble common benign conditions such as blepharitis
- Uncommon (1–5% of eyelid malignancies)
- Margins may be difficult to confirm clinically due to pagetoid spread within conjunctiva, or multifocal origin
- Early diagnosis important
- Regional or distant metastases can occur

Clinical Findings

- Upper eyelid is most common site, most common in elderly patients
- Characteristic findings include thickening of the eyelid and conjunctival injection, which may be confused with blepharitis (Fig. 2.28)
  - Lash loss is possible
  - Ulceration occurs uncommonly (Fig. 2.29A).
- Sebaceous material within the tumor has a yellow appearance (Fig. 2.30)
  - A "tigroid" appearance due to pagetoid spread at the eyelid margin or on the posterior surface of the tarsus (Figs 2.29 and 2.30) can occur
- **Any sebaceous gland in the periocular area can be the source:**
  - meibomian gland (tarsal plate)
  - Zeis gland (lid margin)
  - pilosebaceous gland in the skin, caruncle, or eyebrow

Ancillary Testing

- CT or MRI is indicated if orbital extension is suspected on clinical examination
- Neck and preauricular examination for regional metastases
- Incisional biopsy for suspicious lesions
  - The specimen should be generous, and the possibility of sebaceous cell carcinoma should be discussed with the pathologist
- Sebaceous cell carcinoma can be associated with other adenocarcinomas, especially in the gastrointestinal tract (Muir–Torre syndrome)

Differential Diagnosis

- Blepharitis
- Chalazion
- Basal cell or squamous cell carcinoma

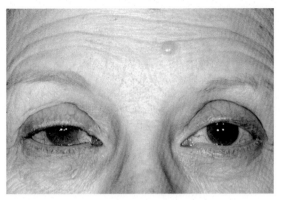

Fig. 2.28 Characteristic findings include thickening of the eyelid and conjunctiva injection, which may be confused with blepharitis.

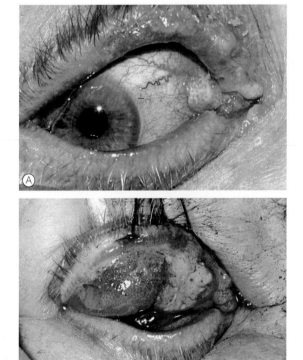

Fig. 2.29 Advanced sebaceous cell carcinoma. (A) Ulceration and lid margin architecture loss with conjunctival spread. (B) Sebaceous material within the tumor appears yellow and may occur in a tigroid pattern at the eyelid margin or on the posterior surface of the tarsus.

Treatment

- No medical treatment
- Radiation therapy can be used as a palliative measure
- Incisional biopsy for diagnosis
- Map biopsies of areas peripheral to obviously involved tissue
  - These biopsies help estimate the extent of any pagetoid spread
- Excisional biopsy with confirmation of free surgical margins, using permanent sections, is necessary
  - Frozen sections are not reliable for evaluation of pagetoid spread
- Reconstruction is performed using standard techniques
- If conjunctival pagetoid spread is extensive or intraorbital involvement is present, exenteration is required

Prognosis

- Cure rate is >90% if margins are free
- Prognosis worsens dramatically if regional metastases present

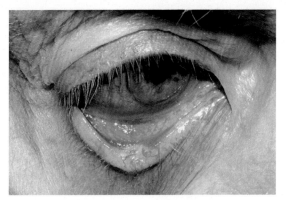
Fig. 2.30 The lesion may start out as a focal area of thickening, often with yellow coloration.

Cutaneous Melanoma

Key Facts

- Malignant neoplasm of pigment cells
  - Rare lesion in the periocular region (<1% of eyelid neoplasms)
- Ultraviolet radiation increases risk
- Early diagnosis important, as regional and distant metastases occur

Clinical Findings

- **Similar characteristics to other cutaneous malignancies:**
  - uncontrolled growth pattern • asymmetric or irregular margins • variation in thickness and color (Figs 2.31–2.33)
- Usually pigmented but can range from depigmented, red, blue, or brown to black—sometimes all in the same lesion (red, white, and blue sign)
- Any pigmented lesion >6 mm in diameter should be considered for biopsy
- **Three pathologic subtypes exist:**
  1. nodular (most common)
  2. superficial spreading
  3. lentigo maligna melanoma
- Cutaneous melanoma may arise de novo or from lentigo maligna
  - Melanoma rarely arises from an acquired nevus, congenital nevi, or oculodermal melanocytosis (nevus of Ota)
- Lentigo maligna (Fig. 2.34) is a brownish patch with irregular borders
  - Neoplastic cells exist superficial to the basement membrane
  - If tumor cells extend more deeply, the lesion is known as lentigo maligna melanoma

Ancillary Testing

- Sentinel node biopsy for thicker lesions
- Metastatic work-up

Differential Diagnosis

- Any pigmented skin lesion, as lesion's appearance can depend on patient's skin coloring
- Benign pigmented lesions appear regular in shape and texture
  - Common benign pigmented lesions are nevi and seborrheic keratosis

Treatment

- Use of sunscreen and sunglasses and avoidance of sun exposure, especially in childhood
- Incisional punch biopsy. Prognosis depends on thickness
- Excision with confirmation of free surgical margins
  - Surgical margins should be wider and deeper than for other cutaneous malignancies
- Free margins are difficult to confirm with frozen sections
  - Permanent sections with fast turnaround time are best
  - Reconstruction is usually delayed pending confirmation of free margins
  - If reconstruction is performed and margins are found to be positive, further resection is required
- Mohs surgical approach remains controversial
  - Evaluation of pigmented lesions using frozen sections is difficult due to artifact
- Standard eyelid and facial reconstruction techniques offer normal or near normal function and cosmesis

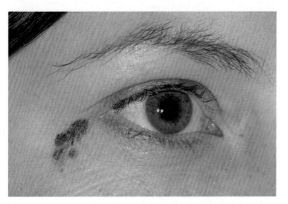

Fig. 2.31 Melanoma arising de novo, with similar characteristics to other cutaneous malignancies, especially those that suggest an uncontrolled growth pattern: asymmetric or irregular margins, variation in thickness and color.

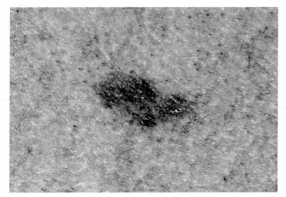

Fig. 2.32 Close-up of a lentigo maligna melanoma, showing variation in color and borders.

Cutaneous Melanoma (Continued)

- Regional and distant metastases are possible even with small melanomas
- Lesions arising from lentigo maligna are difficult to cure locally due to the diffuse nature of the malignant cells

Prognosis

- For lesions occurring away from the eyelids, cure rate depends on depth of lesion
  - Patients with lesions <0.75 mm deep have a 5-year survival rate of 98%
  - Thick lesions carry a mortality rate of ≥ 50%
  - Exact survival statistics for periocular melanoma are not known
- Distant metastasis is more likely than local recurrence, unlike other cutaneous neoplasms

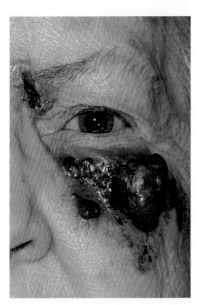

Fig. 2.33 Advanced melanoma. Note basal cell carcinoma near nasal bridge.

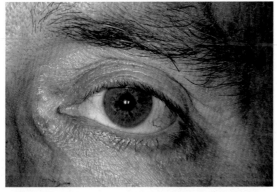

Fig. 2.34 Tan to brown, evenly pigmented lesion with relatively smooth borders, typical of lentigo maligna.

Section 3
Disorders of the Eyelid: Eyelid Trauma

Eyelid Laceration Involving the Margin

Key Facts

- Lacerations of the eyelid margin require careful repair to ensure appropriate cosmesis and function
- **Usually due to direct trauma to eyelid margin, most commonly from:**
  - sports injury • assault • accidental trauma • motor vehicle accidents • animal bite
- Rule out associated ocular and orbital injuries

Clinical Findings

- Ensure that tetanus status is up to date
- Suspect deep penetration into orbit if orbital fat visible
- Consider CT scanning to identify orbital fractures or foreign bodies
- Antibiotics (coverage for gram-positive and anaerobic bacteria) for dirty wounds

Treatment

- Vertical mattress suture, 6-0 silk or 7-0 Vicryl (polyglactin), through the meibomian gland orifices, left untied
- Lamellar sutures in tarsal plate (5-0 Vicryl sutures)
- Additional one or two vertical mattress sutures anterior to the first
- Orbicularis muscle and skin closure
- **Surgical complications:**
  - visible scar • notching of the margin • lid retraction

Prognosis

- Excellent results are common when meticulous closure is performed

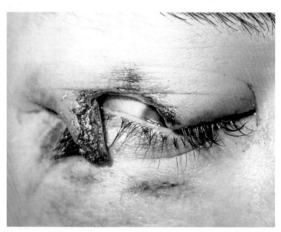

Fig. 3.1 A full-thickness laceration through the eyelid margin.

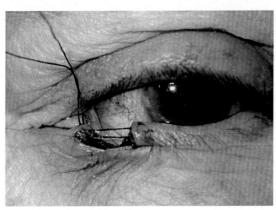

Fig. 3.2 A medial laceration repair with the initial 5-0 Vicryl tarsal suture and initial 6-0 silk margin suture in place.

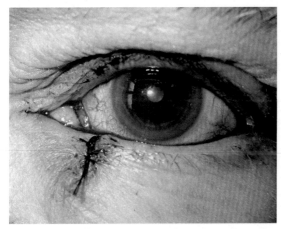

Fig. 3.3 Completed marginal laceration repair.

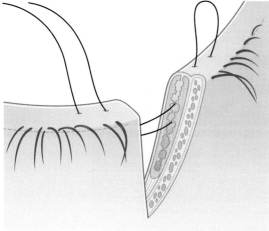

Fig. 3.4 A vertical mattress (6-0 silk or 7-0 Vicryl) suture is placed at the level of the meibomian gland openings. (From Nerad JA 2001 Oculoplastic Surgery: the Requisites in Ophthalmology. Mosby, St. Louis.)

Eyelid Laceration Involving the Canaliculus

Key Facts

- Identification and repair of canalicular lacerations is essential to ensure proper tear drainage system function
- **Mechanism:**
  - sharp trauma to medial eyelid margin
  - blunt trauma pulling eyelid laterally, as occurs with a fist hitting the cheek (may cause tearing of the canaliculus near the common internal punctum)
- **Common periocular trauma, occurring as:**
  - sports injury • assault • accidental trauma • motor vehicle accident • animal bite

Clinical Findings

- Suspect a canalicular injury when there is any trauma apparent medial to the puncta
  - Careful examination is often required to identify a canalicular laceration (see Fig. 3.5)
- Probing of the canaliculus may be necessary to establish the diagnosis
- Must rule out open globe and other intraocular injuries with complete ophthalmic examination
- Most laceration to the canalicular system should be repaired

Treatment

- Ensure that tetanus status is up to date
- Antibiotics (coverage for gram-positive and anaerobic bacteria) for dirty wounds
- Place bicanalicular stents or monocanalicular silicone stent through the lacerated canaliculus
  - monocanalicular or "pigtail" stents are useful with local anesthesis
- Close canaliculus over stents with 7-0 or 8-0 Vicryl (polyglactin) sutures
- Repair medial canthal tendon with 4-0 or 5-0 Vicryl sutures
- Close skin with interrupted absorbable or permanent sutures
- Remove stent in 3–6 months
- **Surgical complications:**
  - visible scar • epiphora • stent prolapse

Prognosis

- Excellent but chronic epiphora possible even with appropriate repair

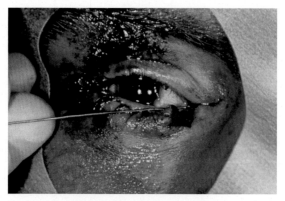

Fig. 3.5 A laceration of the right lower eyelid.

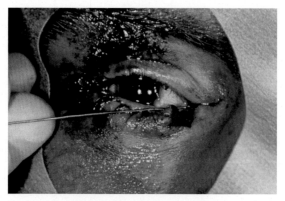

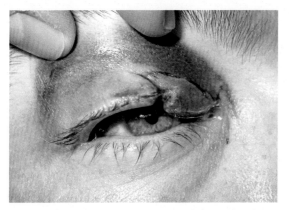

Fig. 3.6 A full-thickness laceration through the midportion of the right upper eyelid as well as a more subtle canalicular laceration medial to the right upper eyelid puncta.

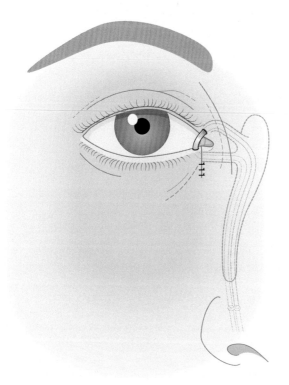

Fig. 3.7 Diagram of the completed repair. (From Nerad JA 2001 Oculoplastic Surgery: the Requisites in Ophthalmology. Mosby, St. Louis.)

Section 4

Disorders of the Eyelid: Involutional Changes

Brow Ptosis

Key Facts

- Descent of the forehead and eyebrows
- Lateral brow ptosis is common, because the frontalis muscle does not extend to the tail of the brow
- Results from collagen and elastin changes, the effects of gravity lead to eyebrow ptosis

Clinical Findings

- Very common in the elderly
- Associated involutional changes of face and periocular area
- May occur due to facial nerve palsy or with trauma to the frontal branch of the facial nerve
- Possibility of brow ptosis repair should be addressed in all patients undergoing upper eyelid blepharoplasty

Treatment

- **Consider goal of treatment:** either functional (due to lateral visual field loss) or cosmetic
- **Consider cause:** paralytic versus involutional
- Multiple techniques are available and must be individualized to each patient
  Direct (supraeyebrow):
    - powerful, straightforward technique • does not address medial ptosis • visible scar
  Midforehead indirect:
    - excellent elevation • addresses medial brow ptosis • visible scar placed in forehead rhytid
  Temporal:
    - can be placed in temporal hair-bearing scalp • corrects lateral droop, not central
  Pretrichial:
    - full lift • improves forehead rhytids • lowers hairline, good for a patient with a high forehead, who does not wear the hair pulled back • risk of hair loss • scar at hair line • scalp numbness • frontal branch injury
  Coronal:
    - powerful elevation • remove rhytids • raises hairline • open approach allows access to frontalis and corrugator muscles • risk of hair loss • scalp numbness • frontal branch injury
  Endoscopic:
    - small vertical incisions hidden superior to hairline • less powerful elevation than coronal • complicated surgery requiring special equipment • risk of facial nerve injury • minimal scarring or hair loss • little scalp numbness
- **Surgical complications:**
    - visible scar (direct, midforehead, pretrichial) • numbness (most common in pretrichial and coronal) • brow asymmetry • facial nerve injury (most common in endoscopic approach)

Prognosis

- Surgical brow elevation provides excellent improvement of brow ptosis

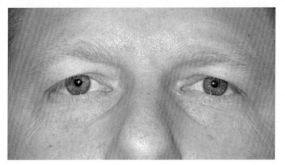

Fig. 4.1 A male patient with brow ptosis and decreased peripheral vision.

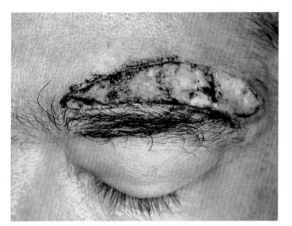

Fig. 4.2 An intraoperative photograph of a direct browplasty.

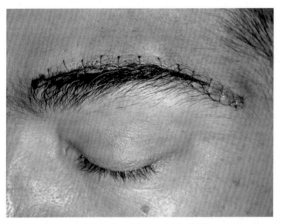

Fig. 4.3 Closure of the direct browplasty incision with a running, locking non-absorbable suture.

Floppy Eyelid Syndrome

Key Facts

- Excessive laxity of upper eyelids, resulting in ocular irritation and conjunctival inflammation
- Possibly caused by excessive rubbing and mechanical trauma, leading to degeneration of tissues of the tarsal plate versus systemic degeneration of the collagen of the tarsus
- Collagen abnormalities of the tarsus have been described
- Exact cause of chronic papillary conjunctivitis and corneal exposure unknown but may be eyelid eversion against the pillow while sleeping
- Most commonly seen in obese, middle-aged men
- **Associated with significant systemic disease, such as:**
  - obstructive sleep apnea • diabetes mellitus • obesity • hypertension • dislipidemia

Clinical Findings

- Unilateral or bilateral red, irritated eyes with conjunctival injection and tearing
- A lax, soft, rubbery upper eyelid tarsus that can be easily folded on itself (eyelid laxity often asymmetric and commonly associated with eyelash ptosis)
  - marked papillary reaction of superior tarsal conjunctiva • mild blepharitis and slightly erythematous skin can occur • other findings include punctate epithelial keratopathy, keratoconus, dermatochalasis, eyelid ptosis, tear dysfunction, and lower eyelid laxity
- **Diagnosis based on:**
  - based on history and examination (suspect in heavy middle-aged men with irritated eyes) • eyelash ptosis (vertically directed eyelashes) often a clue to diagnosis

Ancillary Testing

- Formal sleep studies recommended for all patients to identify possible obstructive sleep apnea

Differential Diagnosis

- Previous trauma

Treatment

- **Medical:**
  - nighttime ointment, patching or shielding to prevent eyelid eversion
    - continuous positive airway pressure for any sleep apnea (may allow patient to sleep supine, decreasing chance of eyelid eversion)
- **Surgical:**
  - full-thickness resection of upper eyelid tissue • the resection can be made laterally or medially • coincident dermatochalasis, ptosis, and lower eyelid laxity should also be addressed
- **Complications:**
  - inadequate resection allowing continued eyelid eversion • failure to address the sleep apnea with associated nighttime eye rubbing and a prone sleeping position

Prognosis

- Surgical treatment is most effective
- Sleep apnea should be treated

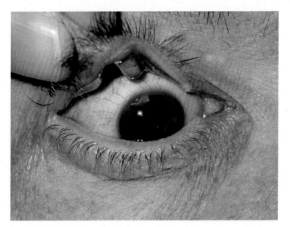

Fig. 4.4 Typical tarsal laxity seen in floppy eyelid syndrome. Eyelid pulls away from globe.

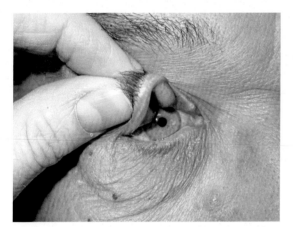

Fig. 4.5 Tarsal laxity often permit "folding" of the eyelid.

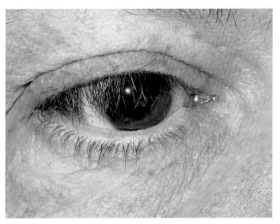

Fig. 4.6 Eyelash ptosis is often a clue to the diagnosis of floppy eyelid syndrome.

Upper Eyelid Dermatochalasis

Key Facts

- Eyelid skin redundancy seen in middle-aged to older patients
- Associated with prolapsed orbital fat giving a fuller appearance to the upper eyelid
- Must make sure eyebrow ptosis is not contributing to this redundant skin
- Determine whether the removal of excess skin and fat is for cosmetic or functional reasons
  - Goal of cosmetic blepharoplasty is to meet patient's expectation in improvement of the eyelid appearance
  - Goal of functional blepharoplasty is to restore a full visual field
- Normal skin fold upper eyelid allows uninhibited eyelid movement and closure, redundancy that must be preserved in blepharoplasty

Clinical Findings

- Cosmetic complaints of loss of normal superior sulcus due to fullness of the fold
  - The upper eyelid crease is not visible, covered with redundant skin
  - Protruding medial or central fat
- Functional complaints of a heavy sensation to the eyelids or hooding of the lateral eyelid (Fig. 4.7)
  - Eyelashes or eyelid skin obstructing the superior visual field; skin can cover the eyelashes (Fig. 4.8)
- Patients often have both functional and cosmetic complaints

Ancillary Testing

- Visual field
- Photographs
- Slit-lamp evaluation, tear function tests for dry eye

Differential Diagnosis

- **Blepharochalasis:** recurrent inflammation and edema to upper eyelid with resultant redundant skin
- Blepharoptosis can coexist
- Brow ptosis can coexist and exacerbate eyelid fullness

Treatment

- Blepharoplasty procedure removes the excess skin, muscle, or orbital fat in the eyelid
- **Preoperative examination should:**
  - identify any associated brow ptosis or blepharoptosis
  - rule out dry eye, corneal disease, lagophthalmos, or lacrimal gland prolapse
- Symmetric eyelid creases (Fig. 4.9) are essential
- Outline an ellipse of redundant skin, leaving identical amounts of skin between crease and eyebrow (10–15 mm) (Fig. 4.10)
  - The remaining skin between the upper mark and the eyebrow must be symmetric
- Excise skin and orbicularis muscle in most cases
  - In the dry eye patient, preservation of the orbicularis may be advantageous
- Determine if any of the two fat pads need contouring
  - Fat removal should leave a small amount of fat anterior to the orbital rim (Fig. 4.11)

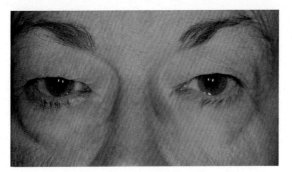

Fig. 4.7 A 67-year-old woman with upper eyelid dermatochalasis. The redundant skin has completely covered the eyelid crease. Eyebrows in good position.

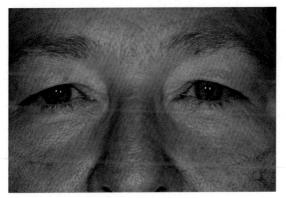

Fig. 4.8 The dermatochalasis is causing the skin of the upper eyelid to rest on the lashes. The patient reported that he can see his eyelashes. This was due to skin causing a mechanical lash ptosis for this patient.

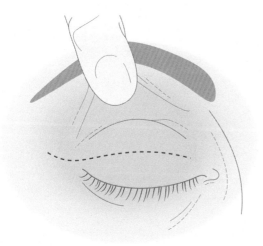

Fig. 4.9 Blepharoplasty marking. Eyelid creases should be marked symmetrically (dashed line).

- The lacrimal gland is located laterally and is lighter in color than the orbital fat
  - If lacrimal gland prolapse is present, the gland should be repositioned in the fossa and sutured to the periosteum
- Closure of the skin can be with permanent or absorbable sutures (Fig. 4.12)

Prognosis

- Excellent—one of the most common surgeries in ophthalmology (Fig. 4.13)
- Must be careful not to remove too much skin from the upper eyelid, which may lead to lagophthalmos and dry eyes

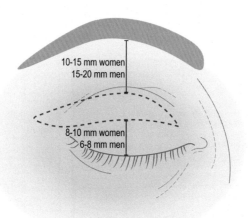

Fig. 4.10 The upper extent of the blepharoplasty incision should be 10–20 mm below the inferior eyebrow margin.

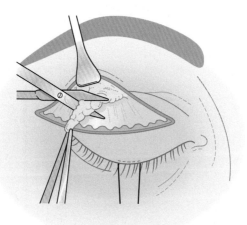

Fig. 4.11 The fat is removed using a cutting instrument of choice. Avoid removing fat posterior to the superior orbital rim.

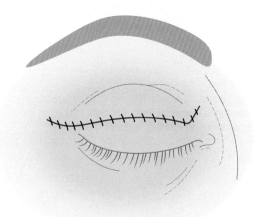

Fig. 4.12 The eyelid incision is closed with an interrupted or a running suture. Before closing, make sure that hemostasis is achieved.

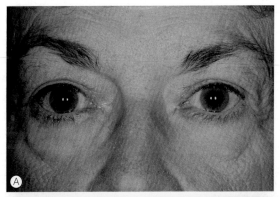

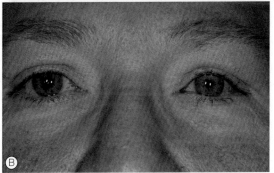

Fig. 4.13 Postoperative appearance of patients seen in (A) Fig. 4.7 and (B) Fig. 4.8. The eyelid crease is visible and the dermatochalasis improved.

Lower Eyelid Involutional Changes

Key Facts

- Includes redundant eyelid skin and wrinkling, eyelid laxity, and fat prolapse descent of the malar fat pad
  - Functional eyelid malpositions, especially ectropion, may be associated
- Patients report that the appearance of the lower lids make their eyes look tired
- Lower blepharoplasty is considered cosmetic surgery
  - In a rare case, the excess skin and fat protrusion may interfere with the patient wearing glasses (Fig. 4.14)

Clinical Findings

- Fullness to the lower eyelid with protrusion of orbital fat (Fig. 4.15)
- Wrinkling of the skin
- Descent of the malar fat pad skeletonizes the inferior orbital rim
  - The nasojugal deepens (tear trough deformity)
  - When viewed from the side, a double convexity forms with the bulge of the orbital fat, deepening at the rim and fullness of descended cheek fat
- Lower eyelid laxity should be determined by one of the following.
  - Snap-back test: the eyelid is pulled down and the lid should reposition itself with one blink
  - Distraction test: ability to pull eyelid more than 6 mm from globe

Ancillary Testing

- Slit-lamp evaluation, tear function tests for dry eye

Differential Diagnosis

- Eyelid edema from thyroid-related orbitotomy
- Orbital mass, which will present as unilateral eyelid fullness
- Look for eyelid malpositions such as entropion and ectropion

Treatment

- Determine which of the three fat pads need contouring before surgery (Fig. 4.17)
  - The lateral fat pad is the most neglected area
- Fat removal alone can be accomplished through a transconjunctival incision
- A cantholysis may be done to facilitate exposure or if the patient needs lower eyelid tightening due to eyelid laxity
- Dissect in the plane between the orbital septum and the orbicularis muscle
- Open the septum to expose fat pads
  - Remove fat anterior to rim (Fig. 4.17)
  - Avoid excessive fat removal in order to avoid hollowing of the lid
- Transcutaneous subciliary incision for conservative skin removal
- **Excess skin removal can lead to:**
  - lower eyelid contour change (round eye) • frank retraction • ectropion
- Blindness due to hemorrhage is a rare complication
- Skin treatment with carbon dioxide laser or chemical peel can rejuvenate the skin and decrease wrinkles (Fig. 4.16)

Prognosis

- Fat removal only often provides satisfying results
- Skin removal need to be conservative to avoid complications

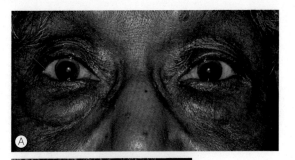

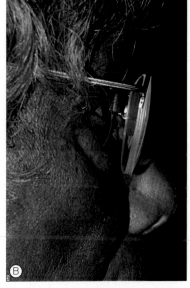

Fig. 4.14 (**A**) Prominent lower eyelid fat pads in an 81-year-old patient. (**B**) Profile view of prominent lower eyelid that almost touches the patient's glasses.

Lower Eyelid Involutional Changes (Continued)

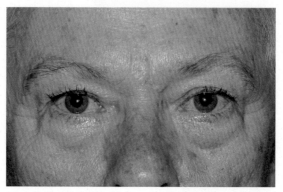

Fig. 4.15 Fullness of the lower eyelid with nasojugal fold demarcating the junction of the descending cheek fat pat and the lower eyelid.

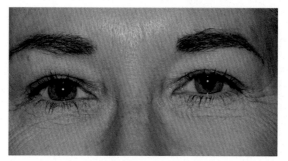

Fig. 4.16 Fine skin wrinkles in the lower eyelids. A blepharoplasty surgery will not eliminate these wrinkles. Chemical peel or laser treatment will improve these lines.

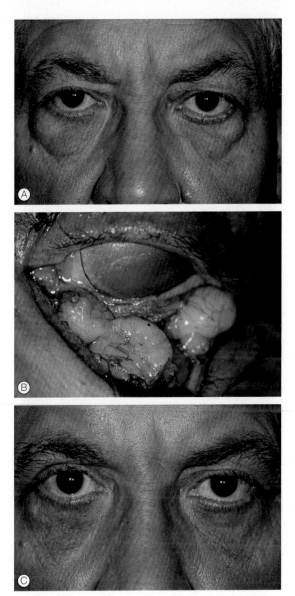

Fig. 4.17 (**A**) Protrusion of the lower eyelid fat pads, with the central and lateral pads most evident. (**B**) Surgical view of the three lower eyelid fat pads after transconjunctival incision. (**C**) Postoperative photograph after lower eyelid blepharoplasty. Residual lateral fat pad remains in the right lower eyelid.

Ectropion: Involutional

Key Facts
- Eyelid margin not be in contact with globe
- Involutional changes result in lower eyelid laxity, primarily lengthening of the canthal tendons, allowing the lid to fall away from the eye
- Common in the lower eyelid of elderly patients
  - Does not occur in upper eyelid
- **Accompanied by other eyelid involutional changes, such as:**
  - ptosis
  - dermatochalasis
  - brow ptosis

Clinical Findings
- All or a portion of the lower eyelid does not rest against the globe (Fig. 4.18)
- Exposed conjunctiva is erythematous, and in chronic cases may be keratinized
- Inferior corneal epitheliopathy is often seen
- Irritation and reflex tearing
  - Punctal eversion can contribute to epiphora, but many elderly patients do not produce enough tears to have true epiphora
- **In unusual cases, the entire lower eyelid may be completely everted:** tarsal ectropion (Fig. 4.19)
  - Consider a cicatricial cause as a contributing factor in this condition

Ancillary Testing
- None

Differential Diagnosis
- Other causes of ectropion should be ruled out, including cicatricial and paralytic causes
  - It is not uncommon to have elements of more than one type of ectropion in a single patient

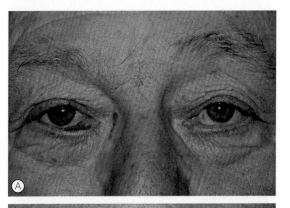

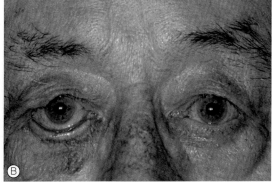

Fig. 4.18 The ectropion may be (**A**) medial, lateral, or (**B**) complete.

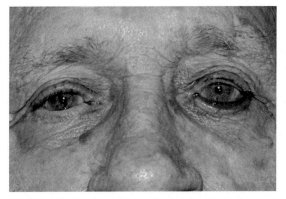

Fig. 4.19 In unusual cases, tarsal ectropion may occur.

Treatment

- Lubrication provides comfort and softens keratinized conjunctiva before surgical repositioning of the eyelid
- Horizontal shortening of the eyelid
  - The most useful techniques shorten the lax lateral canthal tendon and re-establish a sharp lateral canthal angle (e.g. the lateral tarsal strip operation) (Fig. 4.20)
- If the lateral traction on the lower eyelid places the everted punctum into normal position while viewing at the slit lamp, a lateral tarsal strip is sufficient
  - If the punctum remains ectropic, add a medial spindle procedure
- If other factors are part of the cause, other procedures (e.g. full-thickness skin grafting) are used in association with eyelid tightening
- Untreated cases can result in chronic corneal and conjunctival changes
- **Complications of treatment are unusual:** wound dehiscence or late recurrence
- If the medial canthal tendon is very lax, aggressive lateral tightening can pull the punctum too far laterally

Prognosis

- Eyelid tightening corrects symptoms and signs in almost all patients

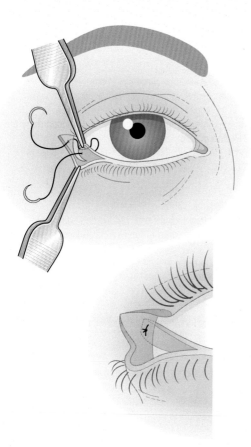

Fig. 4.20 The most common procedure to correct ectropion is the lateral tarsal strip operation. Insert: the strip is placed on the inner aspect of the orbital rim.

Ectropion: Paralytic

Key Facts

- Ectropion of the lower eyelid caused by weakness of the facial nerve
- Loss of orbicularis muscle support causes eyelid to fall away from eye
- Uncommon condition in a comprehensive ophthalmology practice
- **Mild to severe facial asymmetry including the following accompany the ectropion (Figs 4.21A and 4.22A):**
  - brow ptosis • lagophthalmos • incomplete blink • ectropion • shallowing of the nasolabial fold • lip droop

Clinical Findings

- The ectropion may be medial, lateral, or complete
  - Ectropion often worse in elderly patients with pre-existing horizontal eyelid laxity
- Corneal symptoms are common because of the associated lagophthalmos and incomplete blink
  - An intact Bell's phenomenon helps to lubricate the eye (Fig. 4.21B)
- Tearing due to corneal exposure, punctal malposition, or loss of lacrimal pump
- Younger patients may not develop ectropion, because the eyelid is well supported without orbicularis function
  - Any associated loss of corneal sensation (after acoustic neuroma surgery) increases the risk of severe corneal exposure and neurotrophic keratitis

Ancillary Testing

- Work-up for facial nerve palsy should be performed by an otolaryngologist
- **MRI for:**
  - associated neurologic deficit (vestibular symptoms, hearing loss, or cranial neuropathy)
  - progressive palsy over 3 weeks
  - failure to improve within 6 months

Differential Diagnosis

- A work-up should be performed to find cause
  - Bell's palsy is a diagnosis of exclusion, accounting for about half of all facial palsies
  - A postviral inflammatory immune-related cause is suspected in Bell's palsy
  - Corticosteroid and antiviral treatment may be of benefit if given early
- Trauma, varicella-zoster virus, and tumor account for many of the remaining facial nerve palsies
- Surgical trauma may result in either temporary or permanent weakness
  - Repair of a resected nerve with a nerve graft takes ≥ 12 months to heal
  - Recovery is usually not complete

Treatment

- Lubrication using artificial tears daily and ointment at night
- Horizontal shortening of the eyelid, using the lateral tarsal strip, is primary treatment for paralytic ectropion
- For patients with an incomplete blink, gold weight placement (average 1.2 g) (Fig. 4.23)
- **Ancillary procedures (Fig. 4.22):**
  - medial tarsorrhaphy • lower eyelid elevation (with or without spacer)
  - browplasty • midface suspension or sling
- Untreated cases can result in chronic corneal and conjunctival changes

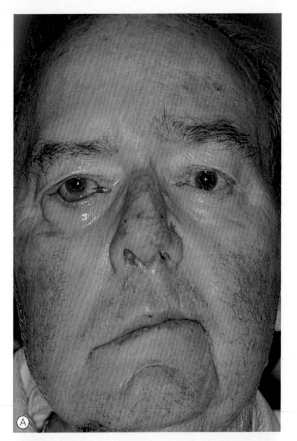

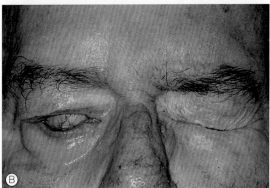

Fig. 4.21 Paralytic ectropion. (**A**) Facial weakness with associated brow ptosis and ectropion. (**B**) Lagophthalmos, incomplete blink, and ectropion contribute to corneal exposure. Strong Bell phenomenon helps to lubricate the eye.

Ectropion: Paralytic (Continued)

Prognosis

- Exposure symptoms can be controlled be a combination of medical and surgical treatment (Fig. 4.22B)
  - Lower eyelid malposition is managed well with eyelid tightening
- Aberrant regeneration of the facial nerve fibers results in facial synkinesis that may mimic an upper eyelid ptosis or may cause eyelid closure with lower facial movement (Fig. 4.22C)
  - Cautious treatment with periocular injections of botulinum toxin (Botox) can improve this

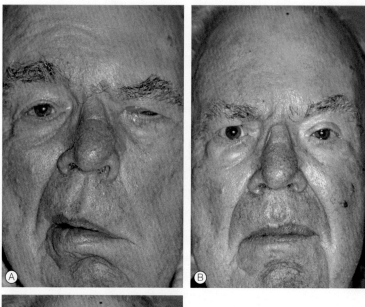

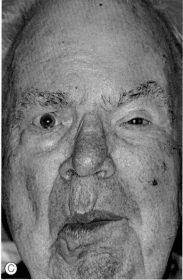

Fig. 4.22 Facial nerve palsy. (**A**) Preoperative. (**B**) After lateral tarsal strip, endoscopic brow lift, gold weight placement, and lower facial sling. (**C**) Aberrant regeneration of facial nerve: eyelids narrow with lower facial movement.

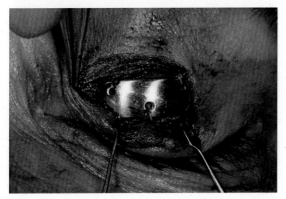
Fig. 4.23 Gold weight placed on anterior surface of tarsus.

Ectropion: Cicatricial

Key Facts

- Eversion of the eyelid margin due to cicatricial process, either traumatic or a skin disorder, which shortens the anterior lamella (skin and muscle)
- A less common cause of lower eyelid ectropion than the involutional cause
- Sun-damaged skin may result in a cicatricial ectropion
  - Basal cell and squamous cell carcinoma should be excluded

Clinical Findings

- Exposed conjunctiva is erythematous, keratinized in chronic cases
  - Inferior corneal epitheliopathy is often seen
- Irritation and reflex tearing
  - Punctal eversion can contribute to epiphora
- **Unlike involutional ectropion, can occur in younger patients with trauma, such as:**
  - thermal burns • chemical injury • lacerations (Fig. 4.24) • Stevens–Johnson syndrome (less commonly)
- Upper eyelid ectropion associated with poor blinking and lagophthalmos

Ancillary Testing

- None

Differential Diagnosis

- Other causes of ectropion (involutional and paralytic)
- May have more than one type of ectropion in a single patient

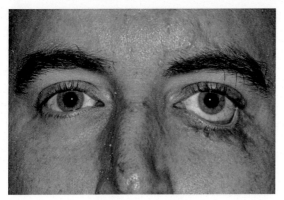

Fig. 4.24 Cicatricial ectropion caused by lacerations after a motor vehicle accident.

Treatment

- Lubrication provides comfort and softens any keratinized conjunctiva before repositioning the eyelid
- If lagophthalmos is severe, the lubricated eye can be covered with plastic wrap at night
- **Surgical repair for exposure due to:**
  - exposure • poor blinking • lagophthalmos
- Aim of surgical treatment is to lengthen the shortened anterior lamella using a full-thickness skin graft
- Definite treatment delayed until the scarring process has matured (6–12 months)
  - Temporizing treatments include lubrication and tarsorraphy
  - Preferred sources of full-thickness skin are the retroauricular or preauricular regions
  - Other sites may be necessary (Fig. 4.25)
- Cicatricial bands are lysed, allowing the eyelid to return to normal position
  - In the lower eyelid, a lateral tarsal strip operation is used to correct any lower eyelid laxity
  - A slightly over-sized graft is sewn in position (Fig. 4.25B)
  - Traction sutures and a bolster secure the graft under a patch.
- Uncommonly, a skin graft will fail or continue to shrink over time (Fig. 4.25B, right lower eyelid)
  - The color and texture of the donor graft may not match perfectly
  - Asymmetry in eyelid position may persist if scarring is significant

Prognosis

- Considerable improvement is possible (Fig. 4.25C)

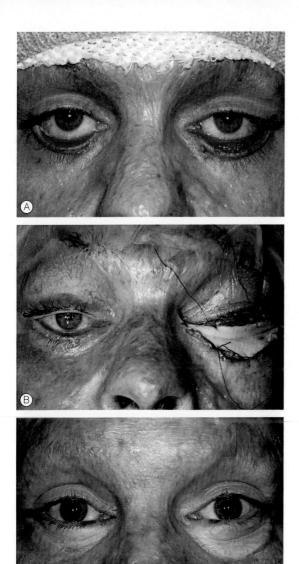

Fig. 4.25 Cicatricial ectropion after thermal burns.
(**A**) Bilateral ectropion. (**B**) Intraoperative view: cicatrix is
released until the eyelid can rest in the normal position.
A lateral tarsal strip operation is performed, and a slightly
over-sized graft is harvested and sewn in position. The
graft is from the supraclavicular region, because of
extensive burns involving more favorable donor sites.
Traction sutures and a bolster secure the graft under a
patch for 1 week. The right lower eyelid has also been
grafted. (**C**) Postoperative view: bilateral full-thickness
grafts had been performed and repeated on the right side
due to shrinkage.

Entropion: Involutional

Key Facts

- Eyelid turning inward against globe
- Disinsertion of lower eyelid retractors, horizontal eyelid laxity, and overriding preseptal orbicularis oculi
- Less common than involutional ectropion
- Increases risk of corneal abrasions and keratitis

Clinical Findings

- **Symptoms may be intermittent or continuous:**
  - ocular irritation
  - foreign body sensation
  - tearing
- **Signs:**
  - lower eyelid rolled against globe with lashes hidden (intermittent or continuous)
  - conjunctival injection
  - punctuate keratopathy
- Diagnosis based on clinical history and clinical observation
  - Entropion may be intermittent and brought out with forced eyelid closure or with blinking in supine position

Differential Diagnosis

- Spastic entropion (associated with ocular irritation)
- Cicatricial entropion

Treatment

- Ocular ointment, bandage contact lenses, or taping are all temporary measures while awaiting definitive surgical correction
  - Treat any corneal infection
- Horizontal lower eyelid tightening (lateral tarsal strip) and reinsertion of the lower eyelid retractors is the most effective treatment procedure
- Everting sutures (Quickert sutures) with or without horizontal tightening can be effective
  - Often done in office but carry a higher risk of recurrence
- **Complications:**
  - recurrence of entropion
  - secondary ectropion
  - eyelid or orbital hemorrhage

Prognosis

- Excellent—recurrences rare with lateral tarsal strip and reinsertion of lower eyelid retractors

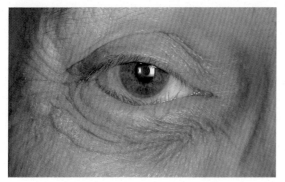

Fig. 4.26 Involutional entropion of right lower eyelid.

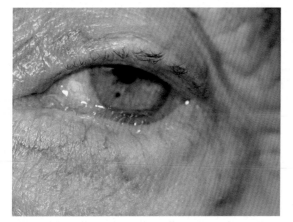

Fig. 4.27 Involutional entropion of left lower eyelid.

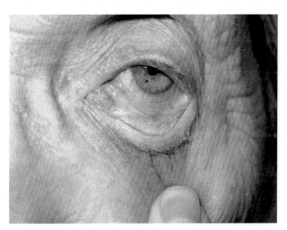

Fig. 4.28 Significant horizontal laxity associated with involutional entropion.

Entropion: Cicatricial

Key Facts

- Eyelid turns inward against globe
- Caused by scarring and shortening of conjunctival surface of eyelid
- **Causes include:**
  - infection
  - inflammatory diseases
  - chemical burns
  - trauma
  - postsurgical
- Relatively uncommon in western world
  - Scarring of conjunctiva due to trachoma is common in other parts of the world
- Increases the risk of serious corneal complications (pannus, scarring, and keratitis)

Clinical Findings

- Ocular irritation, foreign body sensation, pain, red eye, tearing, mucus discharge
- Eyelid margin rolled inward with lashes touching globe, conjunctival scarring and injection, and keratopathy
  - Upper, lower, or both eyelids may be involved
- Diagnosis based on history and clinical observation (cultures or biopsy may be required)
  - Infection: trachoma
  - Inflammatory: ocular cicatricial pemphigoid (biopsy required), Stevens–Johnson syndrome
  - Trauma: chemical injuries, postsurgical (after transconjunctival incisions, chalazion drainage)

Differential Diagnosis

- Spastic or involutional entropion
- **Epiblepharon:** extra roll of skin pushing lashes against eye, normal margin, and posterior lamella
- **Trichiasis:** eyelashes against the eye with normal margin and posterior lamella

Treatment

- Ocular ointment or bandage contact lens for temporary relief
  - Treat underlying condition if infective or inflammatory cause
- **Surgical treatment depends on cause and severity:**
  - tarsal fracture or terminal tarsal rotation–tarsal incisions and rotational sutures
  - direct lash excision
  - mucus membrane or hard palate spacer grafts to lengthen posterior lamella

Prognosis

- Dependent on cause
- Infective and inflammatory causes more difficult than cases related to trauma
  - Related disease process may leave eye dry

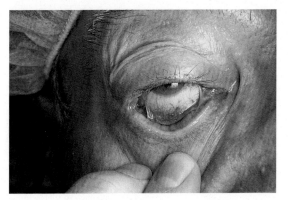

Fig. 4.29 Symblepharon formation in a patient with ocular cicatricial pemphigoid.

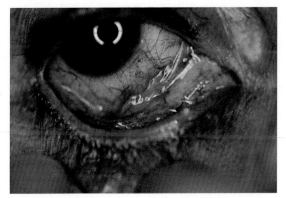

Fig. 4.30 Postblepharoplasty-induced conjunctival scarring causing entropion.

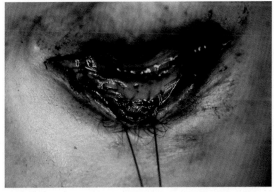

Fig. 4.31 Mucous membrane graft in place in patient seen in Fig. 4.29.

Trichiasis: Marginal Entropion and Other Causes

Key Facts

- Trichiasis commonly refers to any cause of misdirected eyelashes
- Multiple causes (Fig. 4.32)
- In absence of trauma, marginal entropion is most common cause
- Marginal entropion is a subtle inversion of the eyelid margin that misdirects the eyelashes against the globe (Fig. 4.33A)
- Marginal entropion is actually an eyelid malposition, a mild cicatricial entropion
  - Posterior lamellar shortening may be due to chronic blepharitis, previous surgery, or unknown cause (Fig. 4.33B)
- Diagnosis of marginal entropion should be considered in any case of trichiasis

Clinical Findings

- Misdirected eyelashes may occur along a segment or across entire eyelid margin
- Normal eyelashes point in a parallel direction
  - In cases of trauma, the orientation of the eyelashes is typically random
- Most important clue in diagnosis of marginal entropion is position of mucocutaneous junction relative to eyelash roots
  - Because of posterior lamellar scarring, the junction moves anteriorly toward the eyelashes (Fig. 4.33B)
- Posterior lamellar scarring is not obvious
  - When present, the more correct diagnosis is cicatricial entropion

Ancillary Testing

- None

Differential Diagnosis

- Marginal entropion
- Trauma
- Distichiasis
- Epiblepharon
- Entropion, spastic or involutional

Treatment

- Medical treatment of any blepharitis present
- Epilation can temporize
- Tarsal fracture for marginal entropion (Fig. 4.34)
- If misdirected lashes are localized, a wedge resection can be performed
- For lengthy areas of trichiasis, consider excision of anterior lamella containing the eyelash roots
- Cryotherapy and electrolysis are not usually recommended

Fig. 4.32 Causes of misdirected eyelashes: (**A**) normal eyelid, (**B**) marginal entropion, (**C**) epiblepharon, (**D**) trauma, (**E**) entropion (spastic or involutional), (**F**) distichiasis. (From Nerad JA 2001 Oculoplastic Surgery: the Requisites in Ophthalmology. Mosby, St. Louis.)

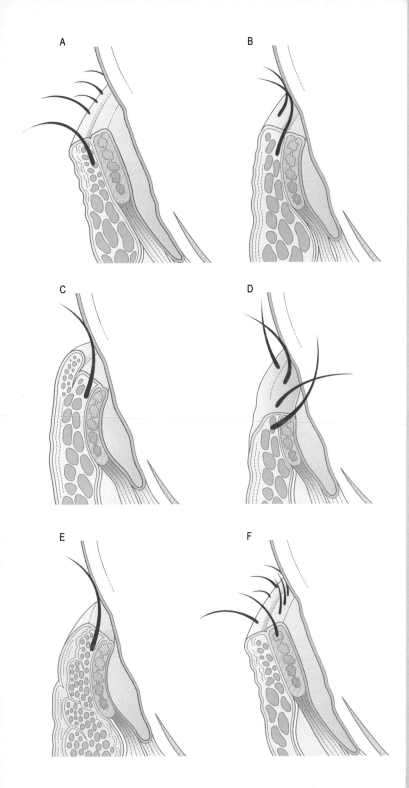

Prognosis

- Excellent—rare recurrence when an appropriate surgical technique is used
- Recurrence is common with epilation or electrolysis
- Cryotherapy tends to destroy eyelid margin

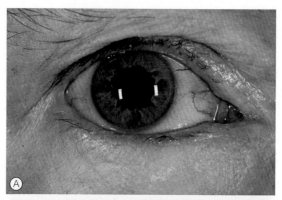

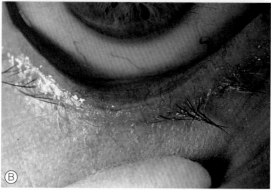

Fig. 4.33 Marginal entropion: (**A**) subtle inversion of the eyelid margin that misdirects the eyelashes against the globe, (**B**) position of mucocutaneous junction migrates anteriorly.

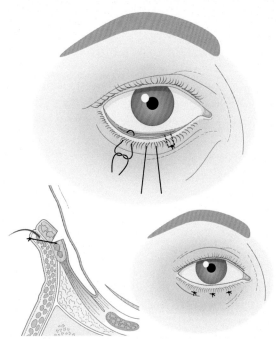

Fig. 4.34 Tarsal fracture procedure. A posterior horizontal incision made through involved tarsus. Everting sutures with 6-0 Vicryl. Sutures tied to evert eyelid margin slightly. (From Nerad JA 2001 Oculoplastic Surgery: the Requisites in Ophthalmology. Mosby, St. Louis.)

Section 5

Disorders of the Eyelid: Blepharoptosis and Eyelid Retraction

Acquired Involutional Ptosis

Key Facts

- Drooping of the upper eyelid occurring with aging
- Most common type of acquired ptosis

Clinical Findings

- Ptosis may be bilateral or unilateral, often asymmetric
- Lower eyelid margin rests on the inferior limbus
- Normal anatomy
  - Upper eyelid rests 1–2 mm below the superior limbus
  - Eyelid fissure measures 8–10 mm
  - Margin reflex distance (MRD) is the distance from the corneal light reflex to the eyelid margin
    - MRD1 is the distance to the upper margin
    - MRD2 is the distance to the lower margin
    - Normal MRD1 is 4–5 mm
- Triad of acquired involutional ptosis
  - High eyelid crease: fibers from the levator muscle to the skin form the crease, so disinsertion or stretching of the aponeurosis leads to the higher eyelid crease (Fig. 5.1)
  - Normal levator function of about 15 mm: when measuring levator function, make sure that the frontalis muscle is not being used to lift the eyelid during this measurement (see *Congenital myogenic ptosis*)
  - Lid drop on down gaze: when the patient looks down, the eyelid remains low compared with the less ptotic side (Fig. 5.2)
- Patients often use the frontalis muscle to elevate the eyebrows and lids in order to clear visual axis
- In down gaze, the eyelid can cover the pupil, so signs and symptoms may worsen with reading

Ancillary Testing

- Visual fields are necessary to document superior visual field loss
- Photographs used to document eyelid position
- Slit-lamp evaluation to rule out dry eye, tearing tests in selected patients
- Pharmacologic testing if ptosis is due to a possible Horner's syndrome or myasthenia gravis ptosis

Differential Diagnosis

- **Other causes of acquired ptosis, such as:**
  - Horner's syndrome
  - myasthenia gravis
  - traumatic or neurogenic ptosis
- **Pseudoptosis from:**
  - dermatochalasis
  - abnormal globe position
  - size (e.g. hypertropia or microphthalmia)

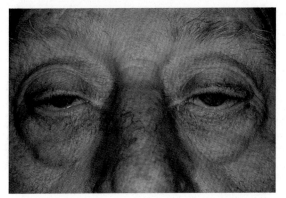

Fig. 5.1 Bilateral ptosis in a 75-year-old man. Eyelid margin is obstructing the margin light reflex. Note the high indistinct eyelid creases.

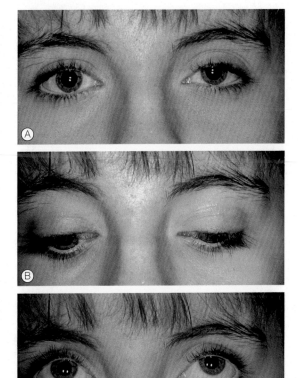

Fig. 5.2 (**A**) Unilateral ptosis of the left upper eyelid in a 27-year-old woman. The eyelid crease is higher on the left. (**B**) The patient is looking down and the left upper eyelid is lower than the right. This is opposite the eyelid lag seen in congenital ptosis due to levator restriction. (**C**) The left upper eyelid moves normally in up gaze.

Treatment

- Levator aponeurosis advancement through an external skin incision is most commonly performed (Fig. 5.3)
- The external skin excision allows removal of excess skin if necessary as part of the ptosis repair
- The levator aponeurosis is advanced and reattached to the tarsal plate (Fig. 5.4)
- Intraoperative adjustments to the levator aponeurosis advancement are based on the eyelid position while the patient is sitting upright and looking in primary position
- Conjunctiva: Müller's muscle resection procedures are used by many surgeons as an alternative to levator surgery

Prognosis

- Excellent restoration of visual function
  - Amount of elevation can be tailored to patient's age and ocular condition
- Can be combined with blepharoplasty and browplasty
  - Significant improvement in cosmesis

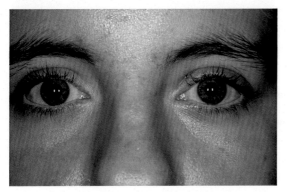

Fig. 5.3 The ptosis of the left upper eyelid has been corrected with a levator advancement. The eyelid crease is more symmetric after surgery.

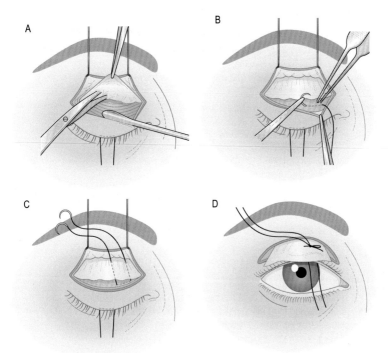

Fig. 5.4 (**A**) The levator aponeurosis is located beneath the preaponeurotic fat pad. It is elevated off the underlying Müller's muscle. (**B**) A double-armed suture is passed through the tarsus. (**C**) Each arm of the suture is passed through the undersurface of the levator aponeurosis, allowing advancement of the muscle. (**D**) The suture is tied in a slipknot and the patient is placed in an upright position to check the eyelid height. Adjustments are made in the advancement to achieve the desired eyelid height.

Ptosis Due to Third Nerve Palsy

Key Facts

- Drooping of the upper eyelid resulting from damage to oculomotor nerve (Fig. 5.5)
- Usually associated with ocular motility disturbance
  - May also be associated with anisocoria
- **Need to determine cause:**
  - vascular
  - compressive
  - trauma
- Levator function may range from zero to near normal
- Diplopia often the limiting factor in treatment

Clinical Findings

- Unilateral ptosis of upper eyelid
- Ocular motility problems depending on division of nerve involved
- Can have inability to move the eye upward, downward, or inward (Fig. 5.6)
  - Usually eye is deviated down and out
- Poorly reactive dilated pupil may accompany
- Vascular causes for oculomotor nerve dysfunction usually do not involve the pupil and recover in 4–6 months
- Bizzare synkinetic eyelid and eye movements may be seen due to recovery by aberrant regeneration

Ancillary Testing

- CT or MRI to rule out a compressive lesion
- Consider an arteriogram if aneurysm suspected
- Fasting blood sugar
- Blood pressure monitoring

Differential Diagnosis

- Compressive lesions such as tumors or aneurysm
- Trauma
- Ischemia
- Myasthenia gravis

Treatment

- Treat underlying vasculopathic causes such as diabetes or hypertension
- Pupil involving third nerve palsy should have immediate work-up for aneurysm or compressive intracranial lesion
- Surgical treatment depends on amount of levator function
  - Good function: levator advancement
  - Poor function: frontalis sling
  - Diplopia needs to be addressed before ptosis surgery

Prognosis

- Guarded, because of the limitation in ocular motility
  - If the ptosis is corrected, make sure that the motility allows for the patient to have single vision in primary gaze
  - Risk for exposure keratopathy is also higher, because of limited supraduction and Bell's phenomenon

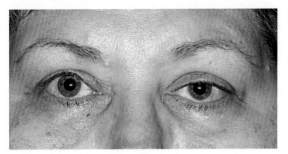

Fig. 5.5 Ptosis of the left upper eyelid in a 46-year-old woman. Note the anisocoria, with the left pupil being larger than the right, consistent with oculomotor nerve palsy.

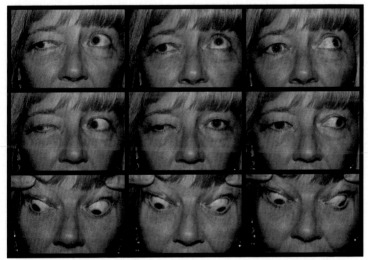

Fig. 5.6 A 52-year-old woman with motility limitations and right upper lid ptosis from a third nerve palsy. Note the marked limited adduction and elevation of the right eye. The patient has less limitation to depression of the right eye.

Horner's Syndrome

Key Facts

- A finding associated with interruption of the sympathetic pathway from the hypothalamus to the orbit
- Usually an isolated finding, rarely caused by an associated carotid aneurysm or apical lung tumor
- Need to localize level in the neurologic pathway at which the disruption occurs (see below)
- Evaluate the patient for other neurologic findings or symptoms

Clinical Findings

- **Classic eyelid position changes:**
  - ipsilateral mild ptosis (1–2 mm) due to the interruption of the sympathetic tone to Müller's muscle (Fig. 5.7) • ipsilateral elevation of the lower eyelid due to paresis of the inferior tarsal muscle (upside down ptosis)
- **Other findings:**
  - miosis (Fig. 5.8) of the ipsilateral side • anhidrosis of the ipsilateral side • heterochromia can be present in congenital cases, the involved iris developing less pigmentation

Ancillary Testing

- Testing based on three neuron pathway
  - Central neuron (first order): from the hypothalamus to lower cervical–upper thoracic cord • Preganglionic (second order) from the lower cervical-upper thoracic cord over the apex of the lung and up to the superior cervical ganglion (Fig. 5.9) • Postganglionic (third order): along the internal carotid to the cavernous sinus and then enters the orbit with the ophthalmic division of the trigeminal nerve, eventually ending up as the long posterior ciliary nerves
- **Cocaine testing to confirm diagnosis:**
  - cocaine blocks reuptake of noradrenaline (norepinephrine) at nerve ending, so more neurotransmitter is available to stimulate the iris dilator muscle • instillation of 10% solution in inferior cul-de-sac of both eyes • normal iris will dilate, but affected iris will not react because of depletion of stored noradrenaline at nerve ending
- **Hydroxyamphetamine testing to localize the defect:**
  - topical hydroxyamphetamine 1% (Paredrine) releases noradrenaline from postganglionic nerve endings • if the pupils fail to dilate, then the defect is postganglionic because the neurotransmitter stores are depleted • if there is iris dilation, a central or preganglionic lesion is diagnosed and a work-up of the neck and lung is necessary • must wait 24 h after cocaine test for accurate diagnosis
- Imaging if second- or third-order defect found

Differential Diagnosis

- Intracranial tumors
- Thoracic tumors
- Aneurysm of internal carotid
- Cluster headaches
- Migraine

Treatment

- Directed at any identified organic cause for sympathetic interruption
- Correction of the ipsilateral ptosis, classically performed with conjunctival Müller's muscle resection, but may be performed with levator aponeurosis advancement operation

Prognosis

- Generally excellent
- **Central and preganglionic causes found with:**
  - apical lung tumors • cranial tumors • aneurysm

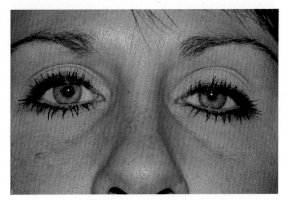

Fig. 5.7 Ptosis of the left upper eyelid in a 27-year-old patient. The left lower eyelid shows minimal elevation.

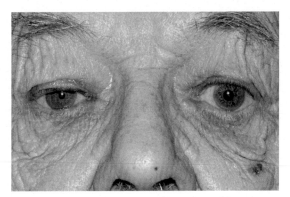

Fig. 5.8 Ipsilateral ptosis of the right upper eyelid, anisocoria, and right lower eyelid elevation in a patient with a right Horner syndrome. The right lower eyelid is at the limbus and the contralateral lower eyelid rest below the limbus.

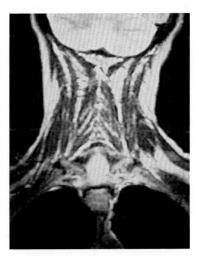

Fig. 5.9 Apical mass causing a right sided Horner's syndrome.

Myasthenia Gravis

Key Facts

- Autoimmune disorder resulting in formation of anti–acetylcholine receptor antibodies
  - These antibodies are present in about 90% of patients with the condition
- Motor end plate receptor dysfunction rendering acetylcholine ineffective, causing muscle weakness
- Can either be generalized (systemic) or ocular only

Clinical Findings

- Unilateral or bilateral ptosis that worsens or fluctuates during the day, typically worsening over the course of the day (Fig. 5.10)
- Involvement of levator muscle and extraocular muscles common in generalized and ocular forms
- Suspect diagnosis in any patient with ptosis and diplopia
- **Cogan lid twitch:**
  - when the patient is asked to look down and then look straight ahead, the eyelid will elevate beyond its natural resting position and then twitch or lower to its resting position
- Motility problems can mimic any ophthalmoplegia condition
- Pupil is not involved with this condition

Ancillary Testing

- **Edrophonium chloride (Tensilon) test:**
  - positive test shows resolution or improvement of ptosis or ocular motility after intravenous administration (Fig. 5.11)

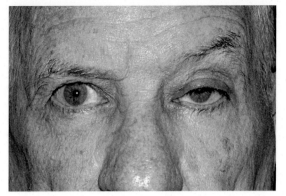

Fig. 5.10 A 67-year-old man with history of fluctuating left eyelid position. Note ptosis of the left upper eyelid.

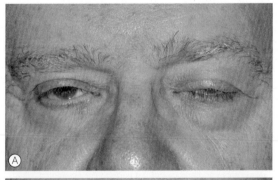

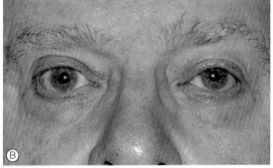

Fig. 5.11 (**A**) Severe bilateral ptosis that is worst in the left upper eyelid. (**B**) Marked improvement in eyelid position after administration of edrophonium (Tensilon).

- **Ice pack test:**
  - ice is placed on eyelids for 2 min
  - the lower temperature improves neuromuscular function and thus ptosis improves (Fig. 5.12)
- **Sleep test:**
  - measure difference in amount of ptosis after 60 min of sleep
  - rest may improve signs and symptoms
- Serology for anticholinergic receptor antibodies
- Chest CT or MRI to rule out thymoma if diagnosis is made

Differential Diagnosis

- Myotonic dystrophy
- Oculopharyngeal dystrophy
- Chronic progressive external ophthalmoplegia
- Third nerve palsy

Treatment

- Medical therapy such as pyridostigmine (Mestinon) to increase available acetylcholine
  - Immunosuppression, usually steroids
- Frontalis suspension after maximum medical therapy has been attempted
- Levator muscle surgery possible, but variability of eyelid position will remain
- Strabismus surgery as indicated
- Thymectomy

Prognosis

- Medical therapy may not be well tolerated because of gastrointestinal disturbance
- Medical therapy may not improve ocular symptoms
- Eyelid and strabismus surgery can improve but not cure ocular symptoms

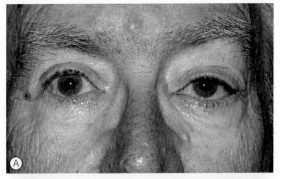

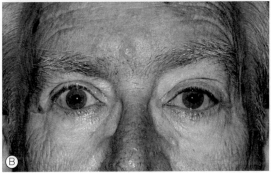

Fig. 5.12 (**A**) Ptosis of left upper eyelid. (**B**) Ice test was performed, with ice placed on the left eyelids. Note improvement in ptosis after application of ice to cool eyelid.

Pseudoptosis

Key Facts

- Eyelid position that appears ptotic but does not measure to have ptosis
- Orbital volume loss or inferior displacement of globe are frequent causes
- Pseudoptosis sometimes mistakenly used as another term for dermatochalasis

Clinical Findings

- Apparent ptosis of upper eyelid
- Often due to loss of orbital volume
  - Frequently manifests as superior sulcus deformity (Fig. 5.13)
  - The high sulcus shows the full vertical height of pretarsal skin, which gives the illusion of a ptotic eyelid
  - May be relative, as when the bony orbital volume is increased in an unrepaired fracture (Fig. 5.14)
- Pseudoptosis may be due to a small globe:
  - phthisis bulbi • microphthalmos • nanophthalmos
- Common in anophthalmos, manifesting as superior sulcus syndrome
- Globe ptosis may produce a pseudoptosis, simulating true ptosis
- May be apparent if there is mild lid retraction of opposite upper eyelid (Fig. 5.15)
- May be result of ocular misalignment (e.g. hypertropia or hypotropia)
  - Make sure you have the patient fixate with each eye separately to evaluate the upper eyelid position
- Redundant upper eyelid skin (dermatochalasis) hanging over the lid margin may be mistaken for ptotic eyelid

Ancillary Testing

- CT scan if fractures suggested

Differential Diagnosis

- True ptosis
- Dermatochalasis

Treatment

- Directed treatment at underlying conditions leading to pseudoptotic eyelid (e.g. upper lid blepharoplasty to improve dermatochalasis)

Prognosis

- Depends on underlying condition
  - Improvements in orbital volume possible with fracture repair or volume augmentation
  - Strabismus, contralateral eyelid retraction, and dermatochalasis can be corrected with surgery

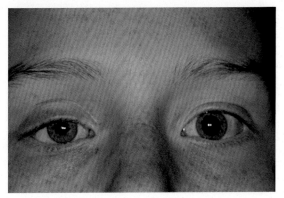

Fig. 5.13 Pseudoptosis of the right eyelid secondary to loss of orbital volume in an anophthalmic socket. Note mild superior sulcus deformity on the right.

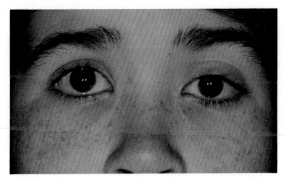

Fig. 5.14 Apparent ptosis of left upper eyelid. Actually, there is globe dystopia with the left eye sitting lower than the right, giving the pseudoptosis appearance.

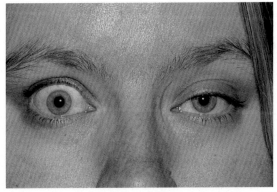

Fig. 5.15 Apparent ptosis of the left upper eyelid. The simulated ptosis is actually due to contralateral eyelid retraction.

Eyelid Retraction

Key Facts

- **Eyelid retraction:** visible sclera between eyelid margin and corneal limbus (Fig. 5.16)
- The eyelid retractors are the levator muscle and Müller's muscle in the upper eyelid, and the capsulopalpebral fascia and inferior tarsal muscle in the lower eyelid
- Normal eyelid position is important for ocular surface protection and normal appearance
- **Most common causes:**
  - thyroid-related orbitopathy
  - inferior rectus recession
  - excessive skin excision during lower eyelid blepharoplasty
  - accidental trauma

Clinical Findings

- Scleral show between corneal limbus and either eyelid margin (Fig. 5.17)
  - The normal upper eyelid rests 1–2 mm below the superior corneal limbus
  - The normal lower eyelid rests at the inferior corneal limbus
- **Increased palpebral fissures:**
  - increased distance from upper eyelid margin to corneal light reflex (margin reflex distance, MRD1) and increased distance from corneal light reflex to lower eyelid margin (MRD2)
- Upper eyelid retraction in thyroid-related orbitopathy often has temporal flare, when retraction is more pronounced in the lateral portion of the eyelid (Fig. 5.18)
- Cicatricial anterior lamellar changes can cause upper or lower eyelid retraction
  - Especially common in the lower eyelid, when associated with eyelid laxity
  - Common occurrence when excess skin is removed during a lower eyelid blepharoplasty
- Ocular surface exposure common, especially with scarring or thyroid eyelid retraction
- Contralateral ptosis can cause eyelid retraction
  - To diagnose, cover or elevate ptotic eyelid and see if eyelid retraction improves
- Variable eyelid retraction results from synkinetic eyelid movements seen with Marcus Gunn jaw winking or aberrant regeneration of third cranial nerve
- Less common causes are congenital retraction and Parinaud syndrome

Ancillary Testing

- CT to rule out extraocular muscle enlargement secondary to thyroid-related orbitopathy
- Thyroid function tests

Differential Diagnosis

- Contralateral ptosis causing a pseudo eyelid retraction because of Hering's Law

Treatment

- Ocular lubrication using artificial tears, ointments, or punctal plugs often relieves the irritation from corneal exposure

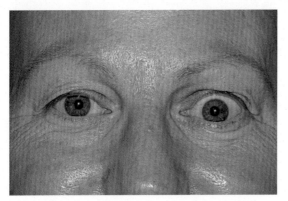

Fig. 5.16 The upper eyelid rests 2 mm below the superior limbus, and the lower eyelid rests at the inferior limbus. The left upper is retracted above the superior limbus.

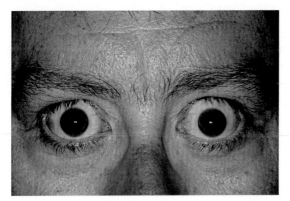

Fig. 5.17 Upper and lower eyelid retraction in a patient with thyroid-related orbitopathy.

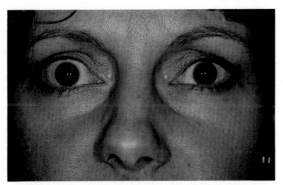

Fig. 5.18 Upper eyelid retraction in 47-year-old woman with thyroid-related orbitopathy. Note the temporal flare of the lateral aspect of the right upper eyelid.

- Recession of upper eyelid, most commonly for thyroid-related retraction
  - Measurement of eyelid retraction should be stable for up to 6 months before eyelid surgery in thyroid-relayed orbitopathy
  - In the upper eyelid, total levator muscle recession and partial Müller's muscle resection
  - The medial portion of Müller's muscle is preserved to avoid medial droop of the upper eyelid contour
  - The recessed levator muscle is secured with hang-back sutures, anchoring it to the conjunctiva, or using a spacer graft between the recessed muscle and the tarsal plate
  - Releasing the lateral horn of the levator muscle is essential to correct the temporal flare of the lateral eyelid and improve upper eyelid contour (Fig. 5.19)
  - Alternative techniques include full-thickness blepharotomy
- Lower eyelid recession
  - Release of eyelid retractors is essential
  - A spacer graft from auricular cartilage or hard palate is recommended
  - Hard palate grafts do not require conjunctival coverage, cartilage does
  - Lateral eyelid tightening should be considered if laxity present
- Retraction from shortening of anterior lamella requires release of scar and lengthening of anterior lamella with a skin graft
  - This is more common in the lower eyelid (Fig. 5.20)
  - Midface lifting may be an alternative technique to correct minor anterior lamellar deficiency

Prognosis

- Excellent if the exophthalmos related to thyroid-related orbitopathy is improved, prior to recession
- Good with eyelid retractor recession surgery
- Skin grafting and spacer grafts well tolerated, if necessary

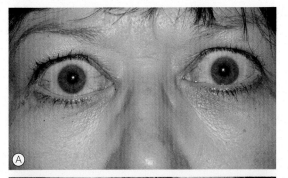

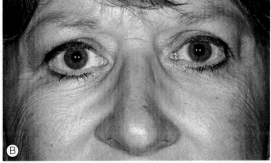

Fig. 5.19 (**A**) Upper eyelid retraction with scleral show in a 57-year-old woman with thyroid-related orbitopathy. (**B**) Improvement in the upper eyelid retraction after levator recession and müllerectomy surgery.

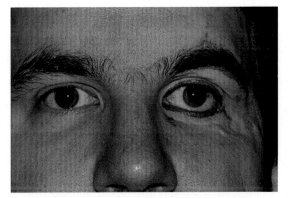

Fig. 5.20 Left lower eyelid retraction after resection of nevus with full-thickness skin graft. The eyelid retraction is from the cicatricial force of the skin graft.

Essential Blepharospasm

Key Facts
- Involuntary bilateral eyelid closure and spasm • A degenerative brain disorder, likely in putamen • Uncommon, occurring in adults >55 years • Spasms are gone during sleep • Botulinum toxin type A (Botox) injections are primary treatment

Clinical Findings
- Excessive blinking is seen early
  - Later, spasm due to over-action of the orbital portion of the orbicularis muscle and the corrugator muscles (Figs 5.21 and 5.22)
- Symptoms vary during daily activities, usually worse when patients are not attentive to a particular activity (e.g. during driving) • Patients develop tricks to keep the eyes open (e.g. placing a finger at the tail of the brow) (Fig. 5.23)
  - Lower face involvement, especially around the mouth, known as Meige syndrome (Figs 5.21 and 5.22)

Ancillary Testing
- None

Differential Diagnosis (Fig. 5.24)
- **Reflex spasm:**
  - various ocular or eyelid conditions can stimulate a reflex spasm • any cause of reflex spasm must be ruled out before facial dystonia is diagnosed • causes of reflex spasm include dry eyes, blepharitis, ocular surface disease, and lid or eyelash malposition
- **Orbicularis myokymia:**
  - fasiculations of one or more fibers of orbicularis muscle only (unilateral, does not close eye, self-limited)
- **Hemifacial spasm:**
  - entire side of face and neck spontaneously contracts • related to facial nerve irritation at exit from brainstem (often more of a spasm than a twitch, cheek and corner of mouth movement easily noticeable, permanent)
- **Aberrant regeneration of facial nerve:**
  - cocontraction of facial muscles that occurs with attempted regrowth of damaged facial nerve fibers • movement of mouth causes narrowing of palpebral aperture, and vice versa
- Consider additional diagnoses of Meige syndrome and apraxia of eyelid opening (Figs 5.22 and 5.23)
- Facial dystonias due to medication uncommonly confused with essential blepharospasm

Treatment
- Botulinum toxin type A is the best treatment (Fig. 5.25)
  - Standard injection of 5 units at five sites
- **Complications of injection are infrequent:**
  - dryness • ptosis • diplopia
- "Immunity" to botulinum toxin is rare
  - Failure of treatment usually due to apraxia of eyelid opening • Patients struggle to open the eyes but have little or no spasm • A frontalis sling of upper eyelid can help the patient to overcome apraxia of eyelid opening
- Surgical "myectomy" can be used if patient is unable to continue botulinum treatments

Prognosis
- Botulinum toxin, repeated every 3–4 months, helps most patients • Essential blepharospasm is a slowly progressive disorder • Surgical treatment not usually necessary

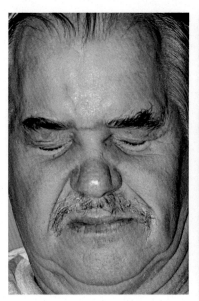

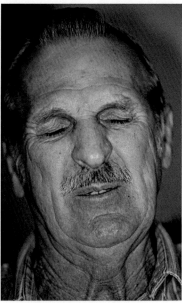

Fig. 5.21 Spasm, due primarily to over-action of orbital portion of orbicularis muscle and corrugator muscles, predominates in essential blepharospasm. Some element of Meige syndrome is present.

Fig. 5.22 Meige syndrome: blepharospasm and lower facial involvement. Note neck involvement in this case.

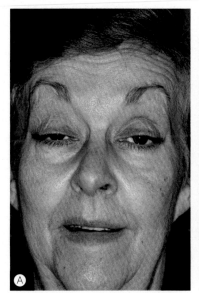

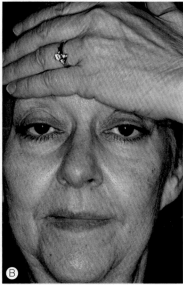

Fig. 5.23 Apraxia of eyelid opening. (**A**) Eyelids do not open and spasm is not present. The eyelids have "forgotten" how to open. (**B**) Many patients discover a trick to keep the eyes open. A common trick is placing a finger at the tail of the brow or holding the forehead.

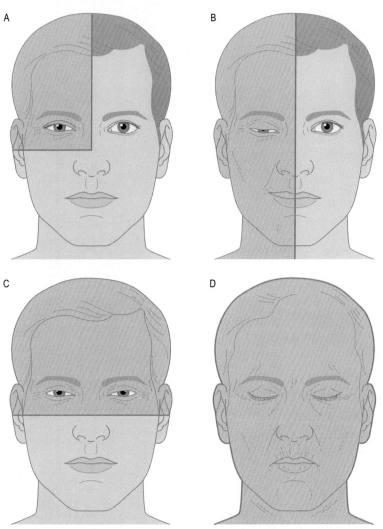

Fig. 5.24 Differential diagnosis of facial movement disorders by quadrant(s) of face involvement. (**A**) Orbicularis myokima: unilateral, isolated to eyelids. (**B**) Hemifacial spasm: entire side of face and neck involved unilaterally. (**C**) Essential blepharospasm: eyelids and brows bilaterally. (**D**) Meige Syndrome: upper and lower face bilaterally. (From Nerad JA 2001 Oculoplastic Surgery: the Requisites in Ophthalmology. Mosby, St. Louis.)

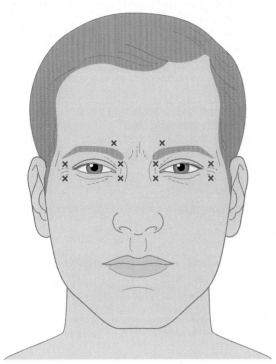

Fig. 5.25 Position of subcutaneous botulinum injections for essential blepharospasm (usually 5 units per site) at five sites around each eye. Improvement in symptoms is expected for an average duration of 14 weeks. (From Nerad JA 2001 Oculoplastic Surgery: the Requisites in Ophthalmology. Mosby, St. Louis.)

Hemifacial Spasm

Key Facts

- Unilateral hyperactivity of facial nerve, causing spontaneous intermittent spasms of the muscles of facial expression
- Unknown cause
  - Compression of nerve fibers may cause axonal damage and stimulate ephaptic impulses (damaged axons excite surrounding fibers)
  - Rarely identified, but vascular compression of facial nerve, as it leaves the brainstem, by a dolichoectatic (tortuous) artery has been identified in some patients
  - Tumors rarely identified
- Uncommon problem
- MRI or magnetic resonance angiography indicated to rule out intracranial pathology

Clinical Findings

- Unilateral spasms of muscles of facial expression, continues during sleep, typically starts in orbicularis and spreads

Differential Diagnosis

- Benign essential blepharospasm (bilateral, not present during sleep)
- Aberrant regeneration of the facial nerve
- **Orbicularis myokymia:**
  - usually due to stress, caffeine, or fatigue
  - uncommonly associated with intracranial pathology (e.g. multiple sclerosis, Guillain–Barré syndrome, brainstem infarction)
- Seizure disorder
- **Reflex spasm:**
  - dry eyes
  - blepharitis
  - ocular surface disease
  - eyelid or eyelash malposition

Treatment

- **Medical:**
  - botulinum toxin injection into the orbicularis muscle is the most widely used therapy (Fig. 5.27)
  - antiseizure and antianxiety medicines used in the past, with limited effectiveness
- **Surgical:**
  - neurosurgical decompression (Janetta procedure), placing a sponge prosthesis between the facial nerve and the offending artery, has been used successfully, sometimes indicated in younger patients
  - myectomy or neurectomy rarely indicated

Prognosis

- Typically, condition controlled with routine botulinum toxin injections
- Rare complete "cure" with decompression surgery

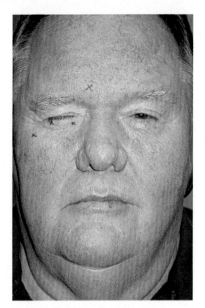

Fig. 5.26 Right hemifacial spasm affecting the eyelids and brow primarily.

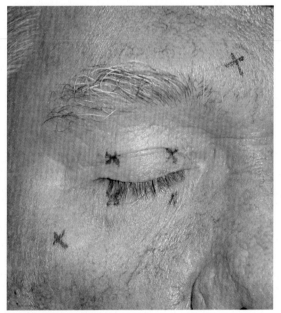

Fig. 5.27 Sites of botulinum toxin injections marked with gentian violet.

Facial Nerve Palsy

Key Facts

- Weakness of facial nerve can lead to serious ocular complications
- Lagophthalmos and ectropion can lead to severe corneal exposure, scarring, or infection
- **Many etiologies:**
  - idiopathic (Bell palsy) • inflammatory • infectious • traumatic • intracranial processes (vasculitis, cardiovascular accident, tumor)
- Common condition
- Facial nerve weakness associated with other neurologic symptoms or signs or a progressive isolated facial nerve palsy demands complete neurologic work-up, including imaging

Clinical Findings

- Foreign body sensation, ocular pain, redness, and tearing
- Paralytic lagophthalmos and ectropion (see *Ectropion: paralytic*), brow ptosis, nasolabial fold flattening, mouth droop
- Corneal exposure ranging from punctate defects to epithelial defects or ulceration (sterile or infectious)
- Diagnosis
  - Bell palsy (idiopathic facial nerve palsy): isolated unilateral facial weakness, 50% of all facial palsies, diagnosis of exclusion, 75% with full recovery in 2 months • May be associated with previous viral infection or diabetes mellitus • Work-up for other causes required for progressive weakness or associated neurologic symptoms or signs

Treatment

- Medical management
  - Based on etiology of cranial nerve 7 palsy, rule out neurologic disease or tumor • Corticosteroids may speed recovery in Bell palsy • Protection of cornea critical • Aggressive ocular lubrication with ointment, taping, patching, or bandage contact lens • Medical tarsorraphy: botulinum toxin injected into levator muscle to induce ptosis
- Surgical management
  Short term:
  - temporary tarsorrhaphy
  Long term:
  - gold weight placement in upper eyelid to improve blinking and closure • lower eyelid tightening to improve ectropion and tearing • lower eyelid elevation to prevent exposure
  Browplasty:
  - for paralytic brow ptosis
  Facial reanimation procedures:
  - include nerve or muscle transpositions • rarely improve blinking
  Static facial slings:
  - can improve cheek, lip, and lower eyelid position • do not improve eyelid closure

Prognosis

- Depends on cause
- **Recovery of Bell palsy is less with:**
  - advanced age • complete palsy at presentation • poor lacrimation • associated hearing dysfunction
- Some degree of aberrant regeneration of facial nerve is common (see *Aberrant regeneration of the facial nerve*)

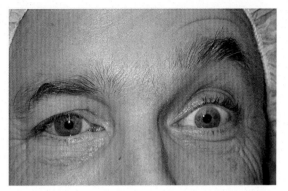

Fig. 5.28 Note inability to elevate the brow in a patient with a right cranial nerve 7 palsy.

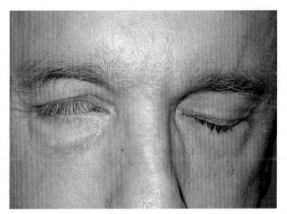

Fig. 5.29 Lagophthalmos secondary to right cranial nerve palsy.

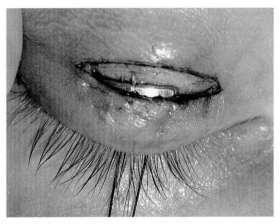

Fig. 5.30 Intraoperative view. Gold weight to improve lagophthalmos.

Aberrant Regeneration of the Facial Nerve

Key Facts

- Abnormal synkinetic innervation of one or more structures innervated by branches of facial nerve
- Most commonly seen as unilateral synkinetic facial movements
- Common after Bell palsy or facial nerve trauma
- Unilateral synkinetic facial movements can mimic hemifacial spasm or eyelid ptosis
- May manifest itself as abnormal tearing or sweating

Clinical Findings

- Ipsilateral narrowing of palpebral fissure with movements of mouth (chewing, smiling, speaking)
  - Test for aberrant regeneration: ask patient to pucker lips and watch to see if eyelid fissure narrows
- These patients may appear to have ptosis because of increased orbicularis tone (look for associated lower eyelid elevation)
- Ipsilateral, synkinetic movement of entire face may appear to be hemifacial spasm, because the whole side of the face may move at once
  - Conversely, true hemifacial spasm is often accompanied by aberrant regeneration (the irritation at the facial nerve root that causes hemifacial spasm may cause nerve injury, leading to aberrant regeneration)
- Uncontrolled, ipsilateral tearing while eating or in anticipation of a meal (crocodile tears)
  - Caused by aberrant taste fibers innervating the lacrimal gland
- Uncontrolled sweating of face while eating (gustatory sweating or Frey syndrome)
  - Seen in facial nerve injury in the area of the parotid gland
  - Caused by aberrant fibers innervating sweat glands

Differential Diagnosis

- Hemifacial spasm
- Orbicularis myokymia

Treatment

- Botulinum toxin injections helpful in controlling facial spasm and any aberrant regeneration
- Botulinum toxin into lacrimal gland may help involuntary tearing

Prognosis

- Can be debilitating but typically controllable with botulinum toxin injections
- Can be functionally and cosmetically annoying
- Typically improved with botulinum toxin injection

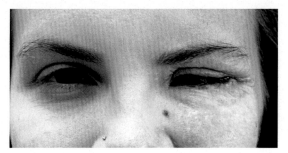
Fig. 5.31 Left-sided facial nerve spasm due to aberrant regeneration after severe facial trauma.

Section 6
Disorders of the Lacrimal System: Congenital Obstruction

Congenital Nasolacrimal Duct Obstruction

Key Facts

- Failure of nasolacrimal duct at valve of Hasner to open at birth
- Tearing or chronic discharge appearing in first several weeks of life
- Unilateral or bilateral, but most are unilateral
- Most will resolve within first year
- Can usually be managed with medical therapy

Clinical Findings

- Children present with epiphora and mattering of eyelids due to chronic low-grade dacryocystitis (Fig. 6.1)
- Epiphora or eyelid mattering may worsen with upper respiratory infections because of nasal mucosa swelling and further duct obstruction
- Acute dacryocystitis unusual but can occur (Fig. 6.2)
- **Diagnosis made by observation of an increased tear lake, especially if:**
  - unilateral
  - mattering of eyelids
  - delayed dye disappearance test (DDT)
- Evaluate for presence of the puncta to ensure that the normal upper lacrimal drainage anatomy is normal

Ancillary Testing

- **DDT:**
  - 2% fluorescein dye is instilled into both inferior cul-de-sacs
  - delay in clearance noted after 5 min (Fig. 6.3)

Differential Diagnosis

- Punctal agenesis or imperforate membrane over puncta
- Canalicular agenesis, stenosis, or obstruction
- Tears arising from lacrimal sac fistula
  - This tearing is different, as it originates from the fistula located below the eyelid on the cheek (may be associated with nasolacrimal duct obstruction)
- Chronic conjunctivitis
- **Reflex tearing due to:**
  - epiblepharon
  - distichiasis
  - other causes

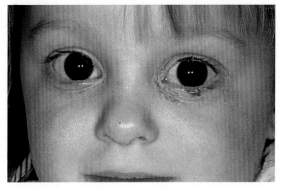

Fig. 6.1 Chronic dacryocystitis: less aggressive bacteria cause a chronic low-grade infection with mucopurulent discharge.

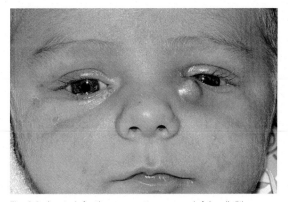

Fig. 6.2 Acute infection presents as a painful cellulitis surrounding the lacrimal sac.

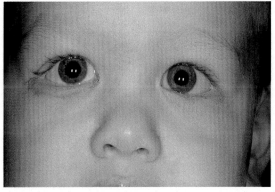

Fig. 6.3 Dye disappearance test.

Congenital Nasolacrimal Duct Obstruction (Continued)

Treatment

- Observation and lacrimal sac massage allows resolution in most patients
- If still symptomatic at or around 1 year of age, nasolacrimal system probing to break the membrane occluding the valve of Hasner
  - Earlier probing if problem is very bothersome
- Probing
  - Probe with a No. 0 or 1 Bowman probe (Fig. 6.4A)
  - Infracture inferior turbinate if inferior meatus is narrow
  - Irrigate lacrimal system after probing to confirm opening of membrane
- For failed probing, place nasolacrimal duct stents
  - Repeat probing and place bicanalicular silicone stents through lacrimal system and retrieve from beneath the inferior turbinate (Fig. 6.5)
  - Monocanalicular stents placed down through valve of Hasner as an alternative
  - Leave stents in place for 3–6 months
- **Dacryocystorhinostomy (DCR):**
  - for the rare case of stent failure
  - for failure of nasolacrimal duct to develop

Prognosis

- Most nasolacrimal duct obstructions resolve in first year
- Probing treats 90% of children who remain symptomatic beyond 1 year
- Probing with stent placement treats up to 90–95% of children who fail probing
- DCR is rarely needed

SECTION 6 • Disorders of the Lacrimal System: Congenital Obstruction

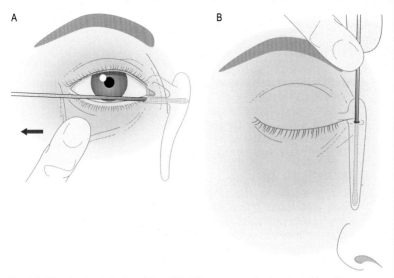

Fig. 6.4 Nasolacrimal duct probing. (**A**) A Bowman probe is placed into the canaliculus until a "hard" stop is palpated. Lateral traction on the lower eyelid helps to prevent "snagging" of the canaliculus. (**B**) The probe is rotated and passes into the nose. Patency is proved by irrigation or direct visualization of probe under the inferior turbinate.

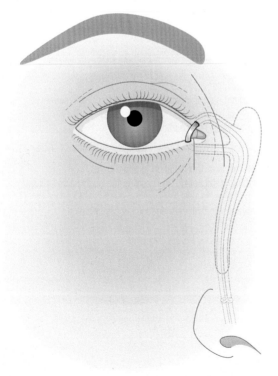

Fig. 6.5 Silicone stents in place. The knot rests in the inferior meatus.

Dacryocystocele

Key Facts

- Mass in medial canthus, present at birth
- Results from nasolacrimal blockage proximally at valve of Rosenmüller and distally at valve of Hasner
- Mucoid secretions distend the lacrimal sac
  - Possibly containing amniotic fluid
- Can resolve spontaneously or require probing
- Also called mucocele, dacryocele, or amniocele

Clinical Findings

- Bluish mass at medial canthus in a newborn (Fig. 6.6)
- Initially sterile but can become infected
- Distention of lacrimal system may extend inferiorly into duct and present with a nasal mass in the inferior meatus
  - This cyst is visible with a nasal endoscope (Fig. 6.7)
  - Because newborns are obligate nasal breathers, these cysts can cause airway obstruction

Ancillary Testing

- CT scan if mass extends above medial canthal tendon, because of the concern of a possible meningoencephalocele

Differential Diagnosis

- Capillary hemangioma (Fig. 6.8)
- Meningoencephalocele

Treatment

- Massage and topical antibiotics
- Probing of the nasolacrimal duct if infection occurs or does not resolve in 2 weeks
- Some surgeons probe at initial presentation

Prognosis

- Lacrimal sac massage can lead to resolution in some cases
- Nasolacrimal duct probing is successful in resolving the obstruction in infants who fail lacrimal sac massage
- Lacrimal duct cysts require removal with endoscopic visualization

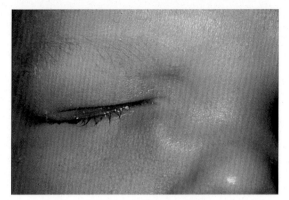

Fig. 6.6 Mass in the right medial canthus in a 4-day-old baby. Note bluish discoloration of the lacrimal sac mass.

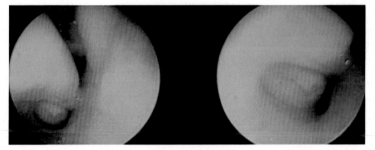

Fig. 6.7 (**A**) Soft tissue mass under the right inferior turbinate. (**B**) Closer view of the cyst that is extending from the opening of the nasolacrimal duct. The cystic mass narrows the nasal passage.

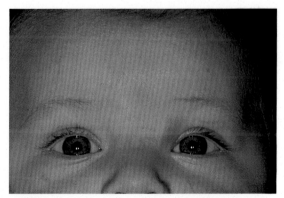

Fig. 6.8 Note the bluish mass in the superior left medial canthus. This represents a capillary hemangiona. It's location above the medial canthal tendon suggests its origin is not the lacrimal sac.

Section 7

Disorders of the Lacrimal System: Acquired Causes of Epiphora

Canalicular Trauma

Key Facts
- Eyelid trauma involving the canalicular system
- Can occur with any facial trauma, blunt or sharp
- The medial portion of the eyelid (canaliculus) is weak and tears easily when lateral tractional forces are placed on the eyelid
  - Fist injuries to the cheek can tear the canalicular portion of the eyelid

Clinical Findings
- Suspect canalicular trauma with any medial eyelid laceration or avulsion (Fig. 7.1)
- Close inspection may be required to identify the lacerated canaliculus
- Probing or irrigation of the involved canalicular system may be necessary to diagnose the injury and identify the proximal cut end (Fig. 7.2)
- Most are avulsion-type injuries from indirect facial trauma
- Occasionally, the canalicular system sustains a laceration from a sharp object

Ancillary Testing
- Probing of the canalicular system

Differential Diagnosis

- Medial upper or lower eyelid injury without lacrimal system injury

Treatment
- Locate the cut ends of the canaliculus using a microscope or loupes
- Repair with pigtail probe and canalicular stent (can be done under local anesthesia) (Fig. 7.3)
  - Place probe through the intact canaliculus around the common canaliculus and out the proximal cut end of the involved canaliculus. The probe must pass posterior to the anterior limb of the medial canthal tendon
  - Thread a piece of silicone tubing 2.5 cm long over a 6-0 nylon suture
  - Place the end of the nylon suture through the eye at the end of the pigtail probe
  - Pull the probe and the suture with the silicone tubing through the cut end and out of the intact canalicular system
  - Dilate the punctum of the lacerated canaliculus and slide the pigtail through the distal cut end of the canaliculus

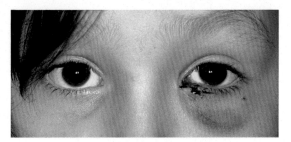

Fig. 7.1 Laceration of the left lower eyelid from blunt trauma that involves the canaliculus.

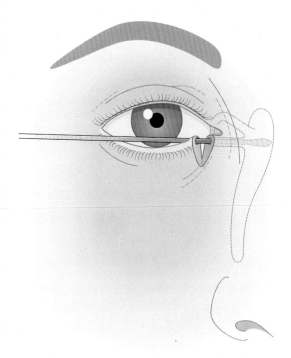

Fig. 7.2 Probing of the canalicular system will locate the proximal end of the laceration.

Canalicular Trauma (Continued)

- Again, place the nylon suture through the eye of the probe and pull the silicone tubing through the normal punctum (Fig. 7.3)
  - Reapproximate the canalicular tissue with interrupted 7-0 Vicryl (polyglactin) suture (Figs 7.4, 7.5)
  - Tie the suture with single throws to close the silicone tube loop
  - Rotate the knot into the lacrimal sac to prevent ocular irritation
  - Repair the eyelid laceration with deep and superficial sutures. No everting sutures are necessary (Fig. 7.6)
- An alternative option is bicanalicular intubation of the lacrimal system into the nose, followed by standard canalicular repair (usually done under general anesthesia)
- A microscope provides helpful illumination, magnification, and a view for the assistant

Prognosis

- One intact canaliculus may provide adequate tear drainage for many patients, especially the elderly
  - However, most surgeons advocate repair of any cut canaliculus
- Repair of the severed canaliculus over a stent usually results in normal tear drainage

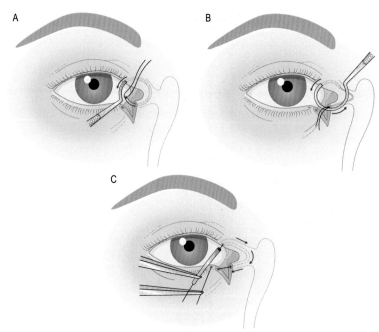

Fig. 7.3 (**A**) Use of the pigtail probe allows intubation of the intact system and location of the distal portion of the lacerated canaliculus. (**B**) The pigtail probe is then rotated clockwise to pull the nylon suture and the silicone tubing back through the lacrimal system. (**C**) The pigtail probe is then passed through the punctum and out the proximal portion of the laceration. The suture and silicone tubing then intubate the entire system. The suture is tied, creating a closed silicone intubation loop.

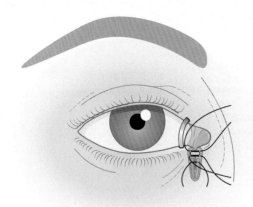

Fig. 7.4 The paracanalicular tissue is closed with 7-0 Vicryl suture. The suture within the stent is tied creating a circular loop of stent through the canalicular system.

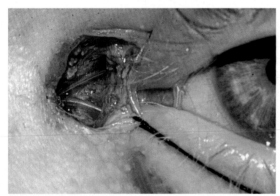

Fig. 7.5 Laceration of the left medial canthus with avulsion of the common canaliculus from the lacrimal sac. The upper and lower canalicular system has been intubated and the next step is closure of the paracanalicular and medial canthal soft tissue.

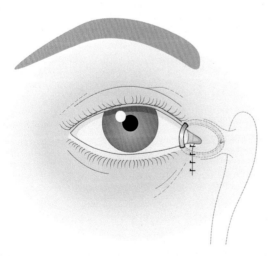

Fig. 7.6 The subcutaneous tissue and skin are then closed.

Canaliculitis

Key Facts

- Chronic infection of the canaliculus, usually presenting as a slight discharge
- *Actinomyces israelii*, an anaerobic gram-positive rod, is most common pathogen
- Uncommon, but canaliculitis should be considered in a patient in whom there is no other cause for discharge
- Under-diagnosed, because often it is not considered in the differential diagnosis
- Successfully treated with aggressive curettage

Clinical Findings

- Discharge
- Swelling and erythema of the canaliculus (Fig. 7.7A)
- More common in the lower than the upper canaliculus
- Occurs more commonly in women than in men
- Pouting punctum is the classic diagnostic finding
  - The punctum is dilated and contains discharge (Fig. 7.7B)
  - Pressure on the canaliculus expresses discharge
- Stones or "sulfur granules" can sometimes be expressed

Ancillary Testing

- Gram stain and cultures are useful for recurrent cases

Differential Diagnosis

- Other causes of discharge (conjunctivitis, blepharitis, dacryocystitis) should be considered
  - Conjunctivitis has more conjunctival erythema, often bilateral
  - Blepharitis shows inflammation of entire eyelid, not just canalicular portion
  - Nasolacrimal duct obstruction can look similar, but pressure applied to lacrimal sac, not canaliculus, expresses discharge, and punctum is usually more swollen

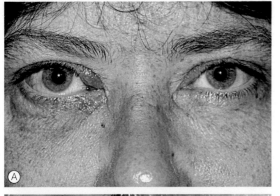

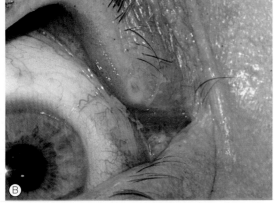

Fig. 7.7 Canaliculitis. (**A**) Swelling and erythema of the canaliculus. (**B**) Pouting punctum is the classic diagnostic finding. The punctum is dilated. This photograph does not show any discharge within the punctum.

Canaliculitis (Continued)

Treatment

- Medical treatment alone is not effective
- Infection situated deep within the canalicular wall
  - Diverticula may be present, filled with granules
- Curettage with a small chalazion scoop should be aggressive enough to clean out all sulfur granules (Fig. 7.8)
- Usually curettage can be performed through the dilated punctum
  - If the punctum is too tight, a one-snip or three-snip punctoplasty can be used to open the punctum
- Curettage should be followed by irrigation
  - Some surgeons use penicillin or iodine irrigation after debridement
- Topical drops, such as sulfacetamide, are used postoperatively
- A wide opening of the canaliculus is recommended if disease is recurrent

Prognosis

- The most difficult part of the treatment is to consider the diagnosis
- Curettage, if done completely, is usually effective
- Recurrences can occur, likely due to diverticula, but are not common
  - Obstruction of the canaliculus may exist preoperatively or may be present postoperatively

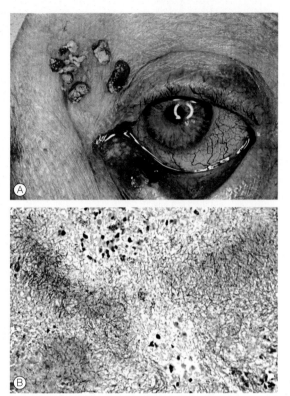

Fig. 7.8 Canaliculitis treatment. (**A**) Curettage should be aggressive enough to clean out all sulfur granules. Three-snip punctoplasty has been performed. (**B**) Gram stain of sulfur granule, showing filamentary bacteria. (Courtesy of Nasreen Syed M.D.)

Dacryocystitis/Acquired Nasolacrimal Duct Obstruction

Key Facts

- Acute or chronic infection of the lacrimal sac resulting from nasolacrimal duct obstruction
- In adults, the obstruction is idiopathic, with scarring of the entire nasolacrimal duct
- In children, the obstruction occurs due to a congenital membranous obstruction at the valve of Hasner
- Nasolacrimal duct obstruction is common in children and adults
- Childhood obstruction usually resolves spontaneously (see *Congenital nasolacrimal duct obstruction*) and does not usually cause acute dacryocystitis
- Adult infections initially treated medically, but the definitive treatment is to provide drainage of the lacrimal sac with a dacryocystorhinostomy (DCR)

Clinical Findings

- Retained secretions in sac become colonized with bacteria
- Acute infection presents as painful cellulitis surrounding the sac (Fig. 7.9)
- Less aggressive bacteria cause a chronic low-grade infection with mucopurulent discharge (Fig. 7.10)
  - Compression of the sac causes reflux of the mucopurulent discharge
- Reflux of material from the sac with digital massage indicates dacryocystitis as a result of obstruction an indication for surgical drainage (DCR) in adults to make the diagnosis
  - No further testing is required
- A mucocele of the sac can result if secretions accumulate in the sac due to blockage of the duct below and at the common internal punctum above (Fig. 7.11)

Ancillary Testing

- The diagnosis of dacryocystitis is clinical
- Irrigation of the lacrimal system is not necessary if reflux with digital pressure is present
  - However, if no reflux is present and obstruction is suspected, irrigation of the system will determine if the nasolacrimal duct is obstructed (adults only; children cannot receive irrigation)

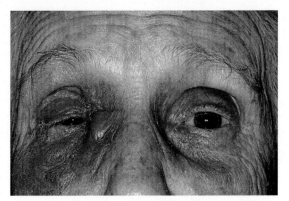

Fig. 7.9 Acute infection: painful cellulitis surrounding the sac.

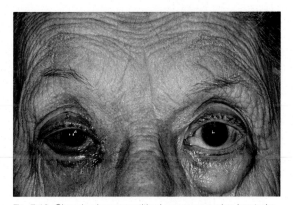

Fig. 7.10 Chronic dacryocystitis. Less aggressive bacteria cause a chronic low-grade infection with mucopurulent discharge. Compression of the sac causes reflux. Ectropion is also present.

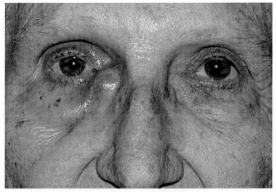

Fig. 7.11 A mucocele of the sac can result if secretions accumulate in the sac due to blockage of the duct below and at the common internal punctum.

- Before nasolacrimal duct surgery, a nasal examination should be performed to rule out intranasal pathology

Differential Diagnosis

- Rarely, a tumor in the lacrimal sac may cause an enlarged lacrimal sac
  - The presence of bloody tears or a mass extending superior to the medial canthal tendon suggests a tumor—CT scan is necessary
- In children, rarely, a capillary hemangioma or encephalocele in the medial canthal area can look like enlargement of the lacrimal sac

Treatment

- Acute dacryocystitis is treated with oral antibiotic therapy, and then DCR (Fig. 7.12)
  - Dicloxacillin or cefalexin (Keflex) 500 mg p.o. q.i.d. for 10 days
  - If an abscess of the sac is present, incision and drainage should be performed
  - A DCR should be done before the time reinfection might occur
- Chronic dacryocystitis is treated with antibiotic drops (e.g. tobramycin) until a DCR is performed
- One episode of dacryocystitis is an indication for DCR
  - DCR should be delayed until after acute infection has been treated
- Complications of medical treatment are rare
  - Unoperated obstruction usually results in recurrent infection
  - Recurrent infections may result in a fistula of the lacrimal sac
  - The success rate for DCR, either endoscopic or external, is >90%

Prognosis

- Once drainage of the sac is established, infection does not recur

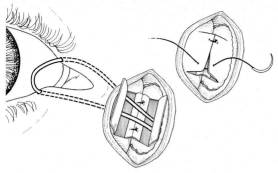

Fig. 7.12 Dacryocystorhinostomy: forms a mucosal lined passageway into the nose. An ostium is created into the nose, posterior mucosal flaps are fashioned and sewn together. A stent is passed into the nose. Anterior mucosal flaps are fashioned and sewn together.

Section 8

Disorders of the Orbit:
Orbital Imaging

CT Scan of the Orbit

Key Facts

- Advances in orbital imaging have dramatically improved our ability to identify and diagnose orbital disease
- In most cases, CT scanning is examination of choice for evaluation of orbital disease
- Ionizing radiation is passed through orbital tissues while a detector records their density
  - Computer formatting and reconstruction software produce planar images (axial and coronal) and three-dimensional reconstructions
- Orbital fat, which has a low relative electron density compared with other orbital tissues, appears black on CT
  - This provides excellent contrast with normal orbital structures and pathologic processes

Indications

- **Orbital trauma,** excellent for visualization and evaluation of:
  - bony fractures • metallic foreign bodies • hemorrhage • emphysema
- **Proptosis or globe malposition**
- **Tumors:**
  - allows identification of calcification, bony erosion, or molding
- **Thyroid orbitopathy:**
  - muscle enlargement • increased orbital fat • apical crowding
- **Inflammatory lesions:**
  - idiopathic orbital inflammation • Wegener granulomatosis • sarcoid
- **Infection:**
  - sinus disease • presence and location of any orbital abscess
- **Preoperatively,** CT scan is extremely helpful
  - Visualizing the bone is important in planning surgical approach to tumors and orbital decompression
  - Repair of facial fractures relies on excellent visualization of orbitofacial skeleton

Ordering CT Images

- Axial and coronal views, 2- to 3-mm cuts
- Bone and soft tissue windows
- **Contrast injection:**
  - helps identify and differentiate vascular tumors
  - not necessary for most orbital conditions or trauma
- Newer machines, which use spiral imaging techniques (also called helical), can complete entire scan in seconds

Risks

- Low-radiation dose, typically 3–10 rads/scan
- Low potential for hypersensitivity reaction to contrast dye

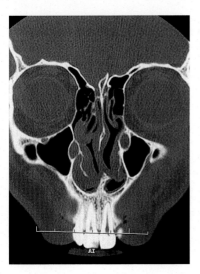

Fig. 8.1 Coronal CT of a patient after facial trauma (bone window). Note the excellent bone detail. There are no fractures noted.

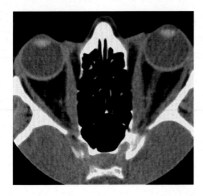

Fig. 8.2 Axial CT showing enlarged medial rectus muscles in a patient with thyroid eye disease.

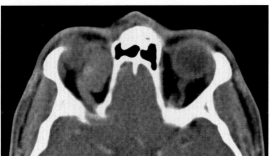

Fig. 8.3 Postcontrast axial CT of a cavernous hemangioma of the medial right orbit. Note the subtle enhancement of the tumor.

MRI of the Orbit

Key Facts

- MRI has limited uses in evaluation of orbital disease • MRI provides excellent soft tissue detail in most parts of the body • However, high signal intensity of orbital fat limits usefulness of MRI in orbital disease • Best for disease at orbitocranial junction (commonly optic nerve)
- **Technique:**
  - protons in target tissue are polarized in magnetic field • protons then excited by radiofrequency pulse and allowed to equilibrate • energy released as protons equilibrate is measured and reconstructed into images • varying pulse and reception time can help delineate tissues in resulting T_1 and T_2 images
    - T_1 images allow visualization of most orbital lesions
- Other specific sequences have been developed to specifically intensify or diminish certain structures
  - Fat suppression makes orbital fat dark, providing contrast for adjacent bright structures

Indications

- Optic nerve lesions, in particular the orbital apex, where high bone density does allow visualization of soft tissues
- Intracranial tumor extension into orbit (e.g. meningioma)
- Orbital tumor extension into soft tissues adjacent to orbit
- **Magnetic resonance angiography can be helpful for:**
  - arteriovenous malformations • fistulas • aneurysms
- Some clinicians, particularly neuro-ophthalmologists, use MRI for evaluation of all orbital lesions

MRI Images

- Axial, coronal, and sagittal images typically provided
- **T_1 sequence:**
  - fat appears bright white, vitreous dark • fat suppression to increase contrast between adjacent tissues • surface coil (energy detector placed on eyelid surface) increases detail • contrast injection—gadolinium–DTPA can help visualize orbital tumors (lacrimal gland and extraocular muscles enhance with gadolinium, optic nerve normally does not)
- **T_2 sequence:**
  - vitreous is bright • edema appears bright, indicating inflammation
- Imaging characteristics of tissues in combined imaging sequences contribute to diagnostic ability of MRI
  - Sphenoid wing meningioma: isointense (with brain) on T_1, bright on T_2, enhances with gadolinium

Risks and Contraindication

- Pacemakers, metallic surgical clips, or suspected metallic foreign bodies
- Claustrophobia while in scanner

Disadvantages

- Higher cost compared with CT
- Longer study time (45–60 min)

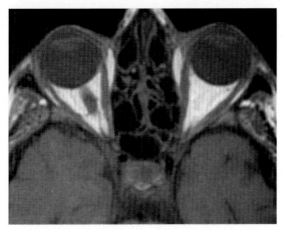

Fig. 8.4 T$_1$ axial image showing excellent soft tissue detail. The vitreous appears dark in the T$_1$ image.

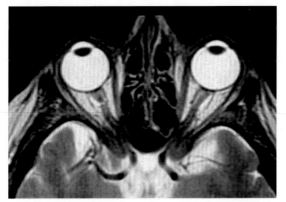

Fig. 8.5 T$_2$ axial image showing the course of the optic nerves. The vitreous appears bright white in T$_2$ images.

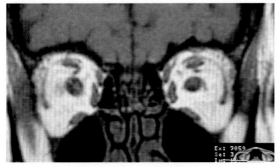

Fig. 8.6 T$_2$ coronal image. Note the optic nerves in the center of the orbit.

Section 9
Disorders of the Orbit: Infections

Preseptal Cellulitis

Key Facts

- Infection of eyelid tissues anterior to orbital septum
- Important to differentiate preseptal from orbital cellulitis
  - Clinical signs: no proptosis, motility change, or vision loss • Source of infection: from cutaneous trauma or adjacent spread (orbital cellulitis usually arises from adjacent sinusitis)
- If symptoms worsen, orbital cellulitis should be considered

Clinical Findings

- Eyelid swelling and erythema limited to periocular area and anterior to orbital septum
  - Eye movements are normal • Pupillary reaction and vision are normal
- Look for evidence of skin trauma (Fig. 9.1)
- In association with upper respiratory infection, suspect underlying sinusitis
- **Sources of infection include:**
  - penetrating trauma • infectious spread from contiguous sources (e.g. impetigo, chalazia, dacryocystitis) (Figs 9.2–9.4)
- Gram-positive organisms most common cause
- Regional lymph node involvement possible
- Local eyelid abscess formation possible

Ancillary Testing

- CT of orbit and sinuses if orbital symptoms occur or if patient not responding to oral antibiotics

Differential Diagnosis

- Orbital cellulitis
- **Tumors:**
  - rhabdomyosarcoma • metastatic orbital tumors • angiosarcoma

Treatment

- Drain eyelid abscess if present, culture for antibiotic sensitivities
- **Oral antibiotics:**
  - gram-positive organisms most common, so penicillinase-resistant penicillin is appropriate
- Hospitalization with intravenous antibiotics if patients do not respond to oral therapy within 48–72 h
- **Incidence of *Haemophilus influenzae* preseptal cellulitis in children has decreased with increased prevalence of vaccination, but keep this etiology in mind if:**
  - the child was not vaccinated • the child is not responding to antibiotic treatment • there is a source for hematogenous spread (e.g. otitis media)

Prognosis

- With prompt use of appropriate antibiotics, these infections will remain in superficial tissues anterior to orbital septum
- Treatment is effective, recurrences are not common, and extension into orbit is rare

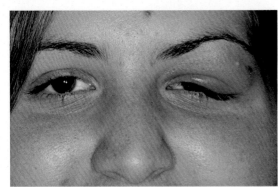

Fig. 9.1 Young adult with diffuse erythema of the left upper eyelid. Orbital examination was normal. Note area that appears to represent trauma site.

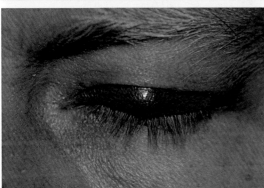

Fig. 9.2 Erythema of the left upper eyelid from inflamed chalazion.

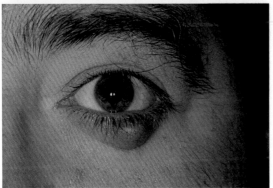

Fig. 9.3 Mass in the left lower eyelid typical of a chalazion.

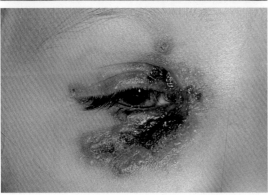

Fig. 9.4 Impetigo of the right periocular area causing a preseptal cellulitis.

Bacterial Orbital Cellulitis

Key Facts

- Acute infection of orbital tissues
- Most commonly occurs in children, usually arising from ethmoid sinusitis
- Penetrating trauma less common cause
- Life-threatening condition
- Potential spread to brain or cavernous sinus
- Vision-threatening condition

Clinical Findings

- Present with marked erythema and swelling of eyelids (Fig. 9.5)
- Pain, limited ocular motility, proptosis, and chemosis (Fig. 9.6)
- Visual acuity usually normal
- Possible fever and leukocytosis
  - Patient appears ill
- In children, often preceded by upper respiratory infection
- In adults, history of sinus disease is common
- **If untreated, can progress to involve optic nerve, with:**
  - vision loss
  - ophthalmoplegia
  - intracranial extension
  - cavernous sinus thrombosis

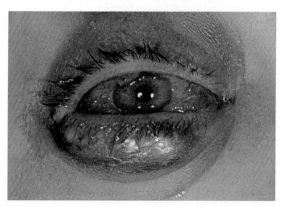

Fig. 9.5 Marked swelling and erythema of the right lower and upper eyelid. Note chemosis and congestion of the orbit.

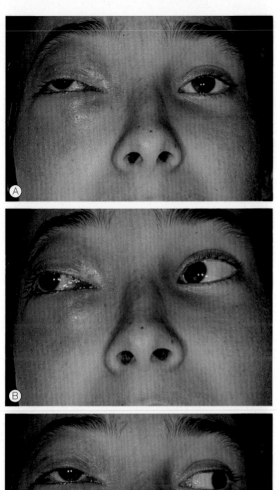

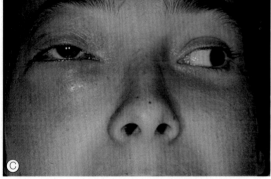

Fig. 9.6 Orbital cellulitis with marked ocular motility restrictions. (**A**) Swelling and erythema of eyelids. The right eye appears slightly higher and more proptotic compared to the left. (**B**) Limited abduction of right eye. (**C**) Even more severe limitation to adduction of the right eye.

Bacterial Orbital Cellulitis (Continued)

Ancillary Testing

- Complete blood count and blood cultures
- Axial and coronal CT views of brain, sinuses, and orbits to make diagnosis and rule out orbital abscess (Figs 9.7, 9.8)
- MRI with contrast indicated if intracranial extension or fungal disease is suspected
- Cultures of sinuses or abscess if surgical drainage occurs

Differential Diagnosis

- Thyroid orbitopathy
- Idiopathic orbital inflammatory syndrome
- **Tumors:**
  - in children, rhabdomyosarcoma, leukemia, and neuroblastoma
  - in adults, metastases
- Preseptal cellulitis

Treatment

- **CT scan orbit and sinus:**
  - if no abscess, hospitalize for intravenous antibiotics
  - if subperiosteal abscess is present in adults, drainage is required
  - if subperiosteal abscess is present in children under age 9 and there are no complications, medical treatment, with close observation, is appropriate; if abscess arises from any sinus other than the ethmoid, or is associated with vision loss, extreme pain, or central nervous system signs, urgent drainage is required
  - Drain any abscess that forms within extraconal or intraconal spaces of orbit
- Treatment team should include ophthalmologist, otolaryngologist, and pediatrician
- Intravenous antibiotics
  Children:
  - gram-positive coverage (**ampicillin sodium–sulbactam** [Unasyn] 100–400 mg/kg per day divided every 6 h)
  Adults:
  - more broad-spectrum coverage (Unasyn 1–2 g q. 6 h). Alternatively, ceftriaxone with or without vancomycin, ciprofloxacin and clindamycin, cefuroxime
- Nasal decongestants can lead to some relief from sinus ostium obstruction
- Clinical evaluations with vision checks are important, especially early in treatment, to ensure that medical treatment is working
- If vision or pupillary changes occur, then urgent reevaluation with CT scan is done and the sinuses and any orbital abscess should be drained
- Increasing incidence of methicillin resistant staph aureus (MRSA) in some communities, therefore vancomycin may be indicated

Prognosis

- Preservation of vision and ocular motility is excellent with appropriate treatment
- Untreated orbital cellulitis can lead to visual loss or death due to cavernous sinus thrombosis or intracranial abscess

SECTION 9 • Disorders of the Orbit: Infections

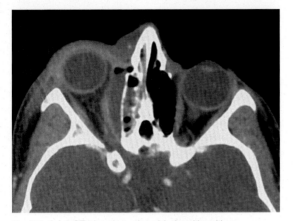

Fig. 9.7 Axial CT showing ethmoid sinusitis with a subperiosteal abscess in the right orbit. Note the medial displacement of the medial rectus muscle and proptosis of the globe.

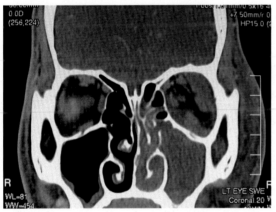

Fig. 9.8 Coronal CT showing opacification of the left maxillary sinus. There is a subperiosteal abscess along the floor and medial wall of the left orbit.

Fungal Orbital Cellulitis

Key Facts
- Fungal infection of orbit
  - Occurs in immunosuppressed patients (see below)
- Lack of normal immune response allows generally non-virulent fungi to invade orbital tissues
  - Vascular obstruction leads to necrosis, the pathognomonic (but uncommon) black eschar in the nose of patients with fungal infection
- Infection arises from inhalation of mold spores
  - The two fungi that cause orbital infection, *Mucor* and *Aspergillus*, are classed in different phyla
- Uncommon
- Difficult to diagnose, because less inflammation than expected is present
  - The most successful treatment is aimed at reversing the underlying immunosuppression, which is often not possible

Clinical Findings
- Typically, a diabetic patient complains of periocular aching
  - Periocular swelling, mild chemosis, and little or no proptosis are present (Fig. 9.9A)
- **Immunosuppression may occur due to:**
  - diabetes
  - chemotherapy
  - drug or alcohol addiction
  - post-transplant medication
- Nasal examination can show mucosal involvement
  - Classic black eschar is seen in only a small percentage of patients
- A chronic low-grade form of non-invasive aspergillus can be seen in healthy patients

Ancillary Testing
- CT scan shows minimal sinus opacification and orbital edema, depending on how immunosuppressed the patient is (Fig. 9.9B)
  - Extreme leukopenia means that the patient cannot form pus
- MRI may show central nervous system (CNS) involvement (Fig. 9.9D)
- Every attempt should be made to optimize patient's general medical status and immune condition
- Stains show fungal elements (Fig. 9.9C)
  - Non-septated hyphae are consistent with mucormycosis, the most aggressive form of fungal cellulitis
  - Septated hyphae suggest *Aspergillus*

Differential Diagnosis
- **Thyroid orbitopathy:**
  - may have eyelid swelling and proptosis but usually bilateral, without pain, and slowly progressive, occurring in generally healthy patients
- **Bacterial orbital cellulitis:**
  - much more inflammation and pain are present
  - CT scan shows significant sinus opacification
- **Idiopathic orbital inflammatory disease:**
  - swelling and pain are much more obvious, onset is more acute, and occurs in non-immunosuppressed patients

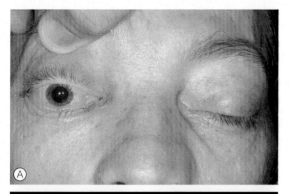

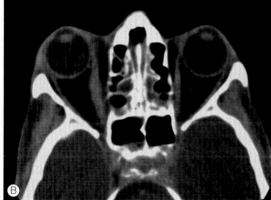

Fig. 9.9 A 44-year-old diabetic man who complained of orbital aching for 1 week. (**A**) Periocular swelling and mild chemosis are present. The patient was leukopenic. (**B**) CT scan shows minimal sinus opacification and orbital edema.

Treatment

- Optimize any underlying medical condition and administer intravenous antifungal medications (amphotericin usually)
- Surgical debridement to remove devitalized tissues
  - Maxillectomy and orbital exenteration may be required
- Hyperbaric oxygen may improve survival, but not proven
- Local packing with amphotericin after debridement may help prevent local spread of infection

Prognosis

- Prognosis is poor in patients unless underlying immunosuppression can be reversed
- Death usually follows CNS spread

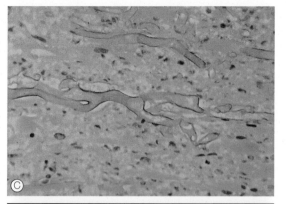

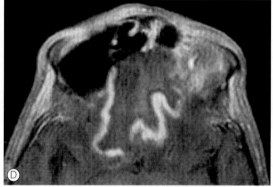

Fig. 9.9, cont'd (**C**) The patient underwent exenteration, maxillectomy, intravenous antifungal therapy, and HBO (hyperbaric oxygen). Exenteration specimen showing non-septated hyphae diagnostic of mucormycosis. (**D**) The patient lapsed into unconsciousness. MRI showing the typical appearance of fungal CNS involvement. The patient died a few days later.

Necrotizing Fasciitis

Key Facts

- Aggressive bacterial infection spreading along fascial planes, difficult to diagnose, treated by wide debridement and antibiotics
- Most common "flesh-eating bacteria" are group A streptococci, less commonly *Staphylococcus aureus* or some anaerobic strains
- Uncommon in periocular area
  - Usually seen in perianal region, trunk, or extremities
- Early diagnosis is best chance of saving tissue loss, vision, and life

Clinical Findings

- Pain and swelling of periocular tissues, a preseptal cellulitis initially
- Initially, infection and necrosis are deep, but eventually the overlying tissue becomes necrotic (Fig. 9.10)
- Extent of clinical involvement based on clinical examination alone is difficult
  - Spread is along fascial planes
  - Look for edema and violaceous discoloration peripheral to any surface infection due to deep tissue involvement
  - Correlate with CT findings in deep tissues
- Often occurs in immunocompromised patients but may occur in immunocompetent patients
- Late involvement may extend into the orbit, leading to visual loss

Ancillary Testing

- **CT scan:** spread along deep fascial planes can be seen (Fig. 9.11)
- Culture and sensitivity of debrided tissues
  - Do not wait for culture results to begin treatment.

Differential Diagnosis

- **Bacterial preseptal cellulitis:**
  - an entry point is usually present, progression is much slower, less deep tissue involvement, much more common
- **Bacterial orbital cellulitis:**
  - usually starts in the sinus after an upper respiratory infection, CT scan shows one or more sinuses opacified, more common
- **Fungal orbital cellulitis:**
  - occurs in immunosuppressed patients so little inflammation present, usually arising from the sinus also, opacification present but less complete

Treatment

- Intravenous penicillin and clindamycin
- Aggressive debridement of involved tissues (Figs 9.12 and 9.13)
  - Involved tissues undergo coagulative necrosis
  - The end point of debridement is healthy, bleeding tissue
  - Multiple debridements are usually required
- Hyperbaric oxygen can be used, but unproven

Prognosis

- Infection can be treated in most cases
- Significant amounts of tissue may be destroyed
- Death occurs in 15–20% of patients

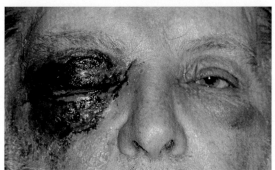

Fig. 9.10 Necrotic periorbital tissue. Edema and violaceous discoloration can be seen in the deep tissues peripheral to the surface infection. Late involvement extended into the orbit, leading to no light perception vision.

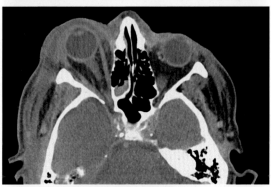

Fig. 9.11 Axial CT: spread is along fascial planes. Note extensive thickening of temporal fascial layers.

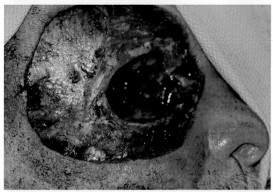

Fig. 9.12 Aggressive debridement of the involved tissues, including fascia under the skin and orbital exenteration.

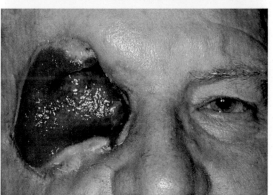

Fig. 9.13 The same patient as in Fig. 9.12 10 weeks after debridement, allowing granulation tissue to form. Note the contraction of the wound. The socket was skin-grafted later.

Section

10

Disorders of the Orbit: Inflammations

Thyroid Eye Disease

Key Facts

- Most common orbital condition
  - Chronic orbital inflammation related to same immunologic abnormality responsible for thyroid gland imbalance • Hyperthyroidism and orbitopathy are known as Graves disease
- Immune mechanism unknown
  - Fibroblasts are targets of inflammatory response • T cell-activated lymphocytes infiltrate tissues, bringing early acute changes • Mediated by cytokine release, free radicals, and fibrogenic growth factors • Fibroblasts are stimulated, causing glycosamine glycan deposition, cell growth, and preadipocyte transformation
- Common, especially in women in the third to fifth decades
  - Five to eight times more common than in men
- Most common cause of unilateral and bilateral proptosis
  - Bilateral extraocular muscle enlargement is seen • Consider in diagnosis of any patient with proptosis

Clinical Findings

- Extremely variable presentation
- **Mild:**
  - irritation • eyelid swelling • conjunctival injection • mild eyelid retraction • corneal epitheliopathy
- **More severe:**
  - proptosis • increased eyelid retraction • restrictive myopathy (diplopia)
- Active and chronic phases
  - Active phase marked by edema and progression of disease (Fig. 10.1A) • Over time, inflammation decreases and chronic fibrotic changes (e.g. proptosis, eyelid retraction, motility disturbances) persist (Figs 10.1B and 10.2)
- Compressive optic neuropathy in up to 5% of patients (Figs 10.1A and 10.3)
- 20% of patients will present with orbitopathy before systemic disease
  - Most patients are or will become hyperthyroid
- Smoking increases incidence and severity of orbitopathy

Ancillary Testing

- Visual field testing to rule out optic nerve compression • Imaging, usually CT scan, to confirm clinical diagnosis • Thyroid function tests (free thyroxine and thyroid-stimulating hormone)

Differential Diagnosis

- Orbital tumors are rarely bilateral
  - If the presentation is mainly unilateral, consider work-up for tumor (lymphoid tumors may be bilateral)
- **Acute inflammation:**
  - idiopathic orbital inflammatory disease (painful)
- **Chronic inflammations:**
  - sarcoidosis • Wegener granulomatosis (mild chronic inflammation associated with systemic disease)

Treatment

- **Mild cases:**
  - lubrication • elevation of head of bed • monitor patients in active phase every 1–3 months
- **Moderate cases:**
  - theoretically control active disease, but no well-tolerated modality • options are pulsed intravenous steroids (methylprednisolone 1 g/day intravenously for 3 days) every few weeks, or alternatively, retroseptal injections of triamcinolone

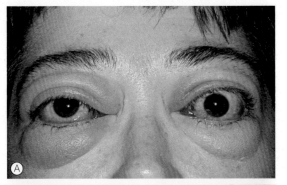
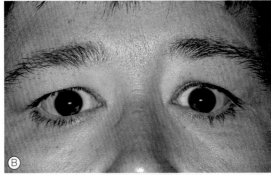

Fig. 10.1 (**A**) Active disease with severe eyelid edema and proptosis in a patient with compressive optic neuropathy (see Fig. 10.3). (**B**) After bilateral orbital decompression, radiation therapy, and strabismus surgery, now in the stable phase before retraction surgery.

40 mg or radiation therapy (20 Gy)—these therapies are controversial • oral steroids cause too many side effects over course of treatment to be useful
- **Severe cases:**
  - steroids (prednisone 60–80 mg/day) to quiet disease before apical orbital decompression • balanced decompression, expanding medial and lateral walls • decompression carries small risk of creating motility dysfunction
- In stable phase, strabismus surgery and eyelid recession procedures
- Untreated severe disease can cause corneal exposure, ulceration, or scarring
  - Optic nerve compression is uncommon but should be ruled out
- Long-term oral steroid treatment causes familiar side effects of steroid dependency

Prognosis

- Frustrating to treat, because there is no treatment to control progression without significant side effects • Patient education, setting reasonable expectations, is important part of treatment plan
- Good vision and comfort can be maintained in most patients
  - Most patients will not require operation
- When needed, improvement in function and cosmesis can be obtained with orbital decompression, strabismus surgery, eyelid recession, and blepharoplasty

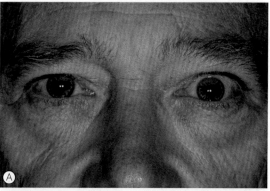

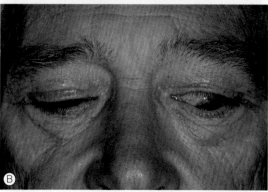

Fig. 10.2 Stable disease with asymmetric presentation. (**A**) Note more proptosis and eyelid retraction OS (left eye). Absence of eyelid erythema and edema puts patient in the stable, inactive phase of disease. (**B**) Lid lag on down gaze typical of eyelid retraction due to thyroid orbitopathy.

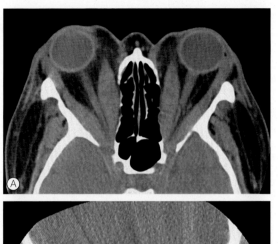

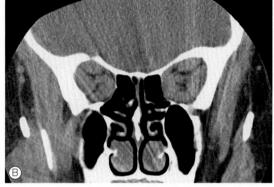

Fig. 10.3 Compressive optic neuropathy: massively enlarged muscles crowding the orbital apex (same patient as in Fig. 10.2). (**A**) Axial CT scan. (**B**) Coronal CT scan.

Idiopathic Orbital Inflammation

Key Facts

- Acute onset of pain and inflammation • Unknown cause • Uncommon • Rule out other cause of pain, CT scan in most cases, then treat with steroids (expecting prompt improvement)

Clinical Findings

- Onset of pain over hours or days • Acute inflammatory findings (Figs 10.4 and 10.5) • Affects all ages, including children
- **May affect any structure in orbit:**
  - lacrimal gland (dacryoadenitis) • extraocular muscles (myositis) • sclera (scleritis) • diffuse
- Must exclude other causes, such as infection or tumor, before making diagnosis
- Response to steroids within hours to 1 day is diagnostic

Ancillary Testing

- Orbital imaging, either CT or MRI, should be performed (Fig. 10.5B)
  - Typically, inflammation extends beyond area of primary involvement
- Biopsy should be performed if presentation is not typical or response to steroid not rapid

Pathology

- **Polymorphic inflammatory infiltrate composed of:**
  - leukocytes • lymphocytes • plasma cells
- Variable amounts of fibrous tissue interspersed throughout

Differential Diagnosis

- **Bacterial orbital cellulitis:**
  - fever • high white blood cell count • malaise • less pain than in inflammatory cases • may have similar onset and progression • CT usually shows sinus disease
- **Thyroid orbitopathy:**
  - slower onset and progression • no pain • sometimes pressure feelings • usually bilateral • less inflammation
- **Tumor:**
  - rhabdomyosarcoma in children • metastatic disease in adults • can have inflammatory signs, but much less pain

Treatment

- Prednisone 60–80 mg p.o. each day
  - An equivalent intravenous steroid dose can be given as an inpatient if pain is severe • H_2 blockers are appropriate to avoid gastrointestinal side effects
- Rapid response expected
  - If not improved in 24 h, reconsider diagnosis, consider biopsy
- Tapering dose of prednisone over 8 weeks
  - Steroid dependency and associated side effects occur
- Symptoms may recur at doses <20 mg
  - Slow taper below 20 mg daily
- Recurrences, sometimes multiple, over time are seen in up to 50% of cases
- For recalcitrant or chronic disease, radiation therapy or other immunosuppressive agents (e.g. methotrexate) have been used.

Prognosis

- Rapid and complete recovery expected in most patients • Recurrent disease that can be very difficult to treat occurs in a small number of patients

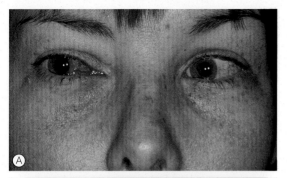

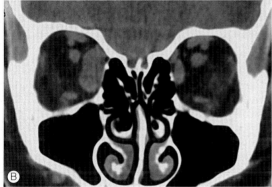

Fig. 10.4 Myositis. (**A**) Typical presentation of inflammation and pain associated with eye movement. (**B**) Coronal CT scan showing enlargement of medial rectus.

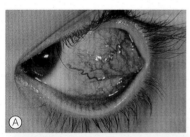

Fig. 10.5 Dacryoadenitis. (**A**) Acute inflammatory findings. (**B**) Axial CT scan showing inflammation centered on lacrimal gland and spilling over to affect surrounding tissues.

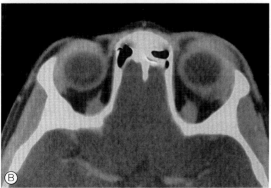

Sarcoidosis

Key Facts
- Chronic granulomatous disorder that causes mild orbital inflammation and/or mass effect
- A disease of histiocytes
  - Non-caseating granulomas are diagnostic
- Uncommon, seen in adults aged 20–40 years
  - African Americans are three times more likely to be affected than caucasians
- **Presents in orbit in one of two forms:**
  - an isolated sarcoidal reaction
  - associated with systemic sarcoidosis (see below)
  - Histopathologically, the two forms are indistinguishable

Clinical Findings
- Slowly progressive mild inflammatory condition
- Eyelid swelling and mild inflammatory changes are seen
  - Involvement of lacrimal gland is most typical presentation
  - Proptosis and lateral ptosis of the upper eyelid are seen (Fig. 10.6)
- Infiltration of any orbital tissue may be present on imaging (Fig. 10.7)
- The sarcoidal reaction is a granulomatous inflammation without any evidence of systemic disease, presenting in the lacrimal gland most commonly
  - 50% of orbital cases are sarcoidal
- Sarcoidosis refers to associated systemic disease
  - Hilar adenopathy occurs in 90% of patients with sarcoidosis
  - Lymph nodes elsewhere, skin, and musculoskeletal system can be affected
  - In orbit, the lacrimal gland is most commonly affected
  - Rarely, central nervous system (CNS) disease may be seen, especially if optic nerve is involved
- **Other ophthalmic findings include:**
  - chronic granulomatous anterior uveitis
  - vitritis (snow banking)
  - retinal vasculitis (candle wax dripping)
  - cataract
  - optic neuropathy

Ancillary Testing
- Serum angiotensin-converting enzyme (ACE) is positive in 60–90% of cases and varies with activity of disease
- Gallium scanning of lung and head (positive ACE and gallium scan increase sensitivity for diagnosis)
- CT or MRI scan of orbit
- Chest x-ray or CT scan
- Orbital biopsy will give diagnosis in orbit and can confirm diagnosis of other systemic findings (Fig. 10.6A).

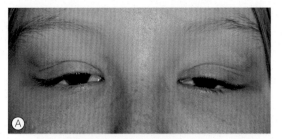

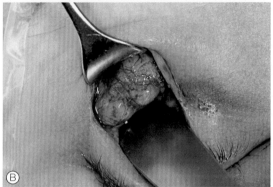

Fig. 10.6 (**A**) Bilateral lacrimal gland enlargement with typical temporal droop of the upper eyelid. (**B**) Anterior orbitotomy for biopsy of the lacrimal gland. Systemic disease was present.

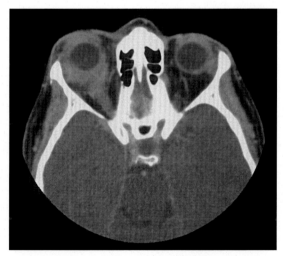

Fig. 10.7 CT scan showing a large orbital infiltrate. Biopsy showed non-caseating granulomas. Systemic disease was present.

Sarcoidosis (Continued)

Differential Diagnosis
- **Other chronic inflammations:**
  - Wegener granulomatosis
- **Chronic granulomatous infections:**
  - tuberculosis
  - histoplasmosis
  - coccidioidomycosis
- **Orbital infiltrations or neoplasms:**
  - lymphoma

Treatment
- Mainstay of medical therapy is prednisone given at lowest dose to control symptoms
- **Other medical treatments include:**
  - methotrexate
  - cyclosporine
  - cyclophosphamide
  - azathioprine
  - more recently, infliximab (tumor necrosis factor agonist)
- No therapeutic role for surgery
- Steroid dependency and associated side effects are part of medical treatment

Prognosis
- Localized orbital involvement (sarcoidal reactions) not thought to become systemic
- Overall prognosis depends on degree of systemic involvement, with pulmonary and CNS complications most severe
  - Mortality rate is 1–5%

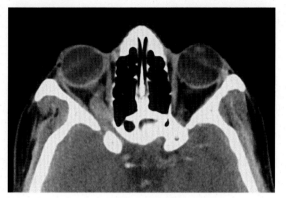

Fig. 10.8 CT scan shows enlargement of the optic nerve. Biopsy showed non-caseating granulomas. Systemic disease was present.

Wegener Granulomatosis

Key Facts

- Granulomatous disorder that can be associated with mild chronic orbital inflammation
- **Mulitsystem involvement includes:**
  - upper respiratory tract • lungs • kidneys
- Unknown cause
- Uncommon but should be considered in differential diagnosis of chronic orbital inflammation
- Histologic hallmark is necrotizing vasculitis
- Serum testing, c-ANCA, useful for diagnosis and to monitor disease activity

Clinical Findings

- Slowly progressive mild inflammatory condition (Fig. 10.9)
- Eyelid swelling and inflammatory changes seen, often bilateral
- Orbital mass or destructive change may be present (Figs 10.9B, 10.10B, and 10.11A)
- **Other signs of Wegener granulomatosis:**
  - oral or nasal ulcers • pulmonary nodules or cavitation • hematuria
- **Ocular involvement:**
  - conjunctivitis • episcleritis • keratitis • scleritis • corneal pannus (Fig. 10.10A) • retinal vasculitis
- The typical saddle nose deformity of the nasal bridge is due to cartilage destruction
- Ophthalmoplegia may be present due to orbital invasion or cranial nerve palsy caused by pachymeningitis
- Neurologic involvement common (22–54% cases)
  - Peripheral neuropathy most common
- Wegener granulomatosis can occur in a limited form without pulmonary involvement

Ancillary Testing

- CT or MRI scan of orbit to characterize orbital involvement
- Systemic evaluation
- Cytoplasmic antinuclear cytoplasmic antibody (c-ANCA) is 98% specific and 98% sensitive for Wegener granulomatosis
- Chest x-ray or CT (Fig. 10.11B)
- Urinalysis to check for hematuria
- Orbital biopsy

Differential Diagnosis

- Other chronic orbital inflammatory conditions, such as sarcoidosis

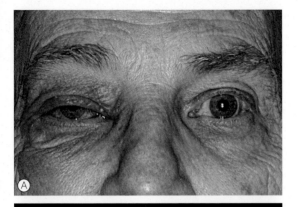
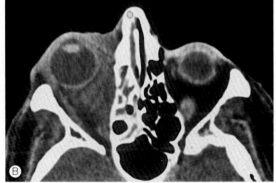

Fig. 10.9 Wegener granulomatosis. (**A**) Chronic unilateral orbital inflammation. (**B**) CT scan: diffuse mass.

Wegener Granulomatosis (Continued)

Treatment

- Prednisone and cyclophosphamide given at lowest dose to control pulmonary and renal effects of disease
  - Methotrexate is an alternative therapy
- c-ANCA level is related to level of disease activity and is used to titrate the dose of medication
- No therapeutic role for orbital surgery
- **Complications:**
  - steroid dependency • associated side effects of chemotherapy

Prognosis

- Orbital disorder causes less morbidity than associated systemic disease
- Overall prognosis depends on degree of systemic involvement
  - Renal failure may cause death

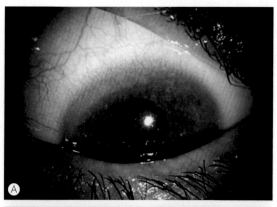

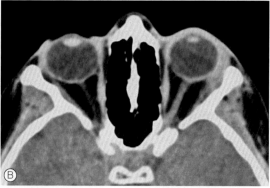

Fig. 10.10 Wegener granulomatosis. (**A**) Saddle nose deformity in 15-year-old. (**B**) CT scan: lacrimal gland swelling.

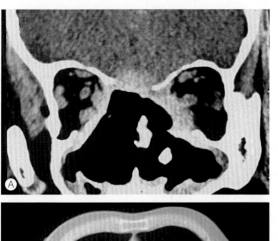

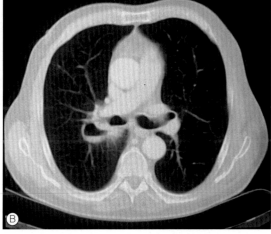

Fig. 10.11 (**A**) CT scan: destructive bone changes with orbital and intracranial extension. (**B**) CT scan of chest: cavitary pulmonary lesions.

Section

11

Disorders of the Orbit:
Neoplasms

Dermoid Cyst

Key Facts

- Round, firm, non-tender mass commonly located along orbital rim, usually suprerotemporal
- Common in children, often appearing noticed after a few months of life
  - Usually diagnosed before age 5
  - Slowly enlarges (Fig. 11.1)
- Arises from trapped embryonic ectoderm within suture lines of orbital bones
- Deeper orbital cysts, often at sphenozygomatic suture line, may present later in life as painless proptosis

Clinical Findings

- **Diagnosis usually clinical:**
  - painless, palpable, round, firm mass located along orbital rim
- Most commonly arising at frontozygomatic suture
  - Less commonly, frontonasal or frontolacrimal suture
- May present with inflammatory symptoms if cyst ruptures

Imaging

- **CT scan indicated if:**
  - orbital extension through suture line is suspected (dumbbell dermoid)
  - diagnosis is in doubt
  - proptosis is present
- CT shows round, well-defined, thin-walled cystic structure
  - Contents usually have fat density (Fig. 11.2)
  - Occasionally, a fat–soft tissue interface will be present, suggesting presence of hair in the cyst
  - Fossa formation is common (up to 75%)

Pathology

- Thin-walled cyst with dermal and epidermal elements in lumen
  - Some cysts have only epidermal elements present (epidermoid cyst)

Differential Diagnosis

- Conjunctival cyst, epidermal inclusion cyst, teratoma, hematic cyst, hydrocystoma, mucocele, encephalocele

Treatment

- Complete surgical excision with intact capsule
- Rupture of cyst may result in significant tissue reaction

Prognosis

- Excellent
  - Recurrences are rare but may occur, especially if cyst is ruptured

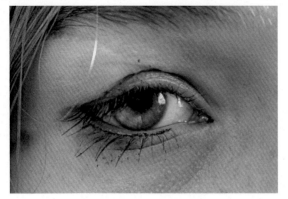

Fig. 11.1 A cyst arising at the frontozygomatic suture along the right superior lateral orbital rim.

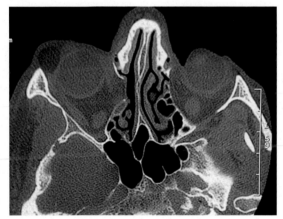

Fig. 11.2 A CT scan of a right orbital dermoid cyst.

Lipodermoid

Key Facts

- Benign, congenital choristoma of collagenous connective tissue and fat located on bulbar surface of the globe, often extending into the orbit
- Choristoma is defined as a proliferation of normal tissue in an abnormal location
- Idiopathic, often seen in syndromic children
- Uncommon, overall, but seen in half of Goldenhar syndrome patients

Clinical Findings

- Elevated, smooth, pink, white, or yellowish bulbar mass
- Most temporal, can be unilateral or bilateral
- Varies from small to bulky tumors filling the palpebral fissure
- **May lead to:**
  - corneal exposure
  - astigmatism
  - amblyopia
- Histopathologically consists of abnormally dense stroma with large deposits of fat covered in keratinized epithelium

Imaging

- Rarely indicated

Differential Diagnosis

- **Prolapsed orbital fat:**
  - more yellow
  - less firm
  - can prolapse with pressure on globe
  - uncommon in children
- **Other choristomas include:**
  - limbal dermoids
  - teratomas
  - epidermoid and dermoid cysts

Treatment

- **Medical:**
  - observation of small lesions
  - removal if astigmatism or amblyopia present
- **Surgical:**
  - lamellar dissection of sclera and/or cornea and excision of visible lesion
  - excision of orbital extension rarely indicated, may damage muscle or lacrimal gland
  - complete removal frequently impossible and not required for appropriate improvement
  - lamellar keratoplasty may be required to deal with any corneal opacity from lesions encroaching on visual axis

Prognosis

- Good
  - Recurrences do not occur

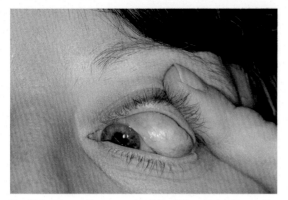

Fig. 11.3 A larger lipodermoid of the left superior temporal orbit.

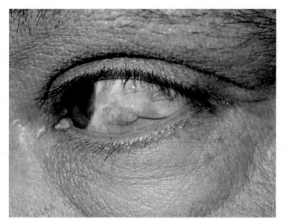

Fig. 11.4 A lipodermoid confined to the bulbar surface of the left eye.

Capillary Hemangioma

Key Facts

- Most common vascular orbital and periorbital tumor in children
- Unknown cause, possibly exuberant mast cell activity or hamartomatous origin
- Very common (1–2% of newborns have lesions on some part of the body)
- 5% of lesions are solely intraorbital, with proptosis and globe displacement and no cutaneous signs
  - Amblyopia may develop due to ptosis, strabismus, or anisometropia

Clinical Findings

- Diagnosis typically made by clinical examination
- Bright red or maroon strawberry mark on eyelid or periocular skin
  - Deeper lesions may appear only as swollen eyelid
- Noted in first month of life, grows to maximum size in 12–18 months, size stabilizes, spontaneous involution by 8 years
- Histopathologically consists of benign proliferation of endothelial cells

Imaging

- CT or MRI not usually indicated
  - For deeper orbital lesions, imaging shows infiltrating non-encapsulated mass conforming to surrounding orbital structures
- Enhances with contrast
- No bony erosion
- Orbital expansion may be present in larger lesions, suggesting in utero formation

Differential Diagnosis

- Lymphangioma most common
- Encephalocele if deep and medial

Treatment

- Check for amblyopia due to occlusion or astigmatism
- Check for orbital dystopia if there is a large orbital component
- Observe for lesions not affecting vision or orbital development for regression over time
- **Medical:**
  - intralesional injections of short- and long-acting corticosteroids for isolated lesions, rare central retinal artery emboli reported
  - systemic corticosteroids for large, diffuse, or orbital lesions (systemic adrenal suppression possible)
- **Surgical:**
  - careful surgical debulking in rare cases
  - laser therapy may be useful for small lesions or residual vessels after involution

Prognosis

- Most patients do well
- Depends on location (orbital lesions have worse prognosis)
  - Amblyopia therapy may be required
  - Facial deformity, usually globe ptosis, can occur with large lesions
- Spontaneous regression in 30% by 3 years, 50% by 5 years, and 90% by 7 years of age
- Residual skin changes may be improved with surgery, laser, or makeup

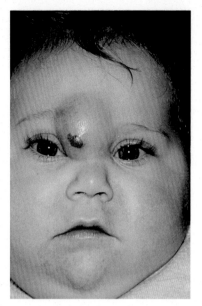

Fig. 11.5 Capillary hemangioma of the glabellar area.

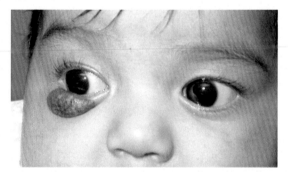

Fig. 11.6 Capillary hemangioma of the right lower eyelid.

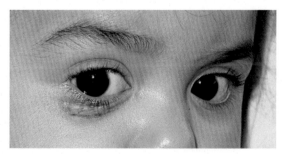

Fig. 11.7 Same lesion as in Fig. 11.6 6 months after corticosteroid injection.

Cavernous Hemangioma

Key Facts

- Most common benign primary orbital neoplasm in adults
  - About 4% of all orbital tumors
- Unknown cause
  - May be a congenital hamartoma of vascular origin
- Typically intraconal, producing axial proptosis
- Usually presents at age 30–50 years
- Often discovered as incidental finding on imaging for other conditions

Clinical Findings

- Painless, slowly progressive proptosis over many years
- Typically unilateral
- Visual loss uncommon
- Found in adults, more common in women
- Encapsulated tumor composed of multiple large, blood-filled channels lined by flattened endothelial cells

Imaging

- CT or MRI shows a discrete round or oval mass without inflammation or infiltration of surrounding tissues
  - 88% are intraconal

Differential Diagnosis

- **Other round isolated orbital tumors or cysts:**
  - schwannoma
  - neurolemmoma
  - dermoid cyst

Treatment

- If asymptomatic and discovered incidentally, many are observed
- **Complete surgical excision of tumor indicated for:**
  - bothersome proptosis
  - diplopia (uncommon)
  - visual changes due to apical compression or choroidal folds (uncommon)

Prognosis

- Excellent with complete resection
  - Recurrences rare

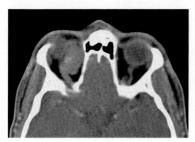

Fig. 11.8 CT scan with a well-circumscribed lesion in the right orbit.

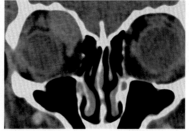

Fig. 11.9 Another example of a right orbit lesion.

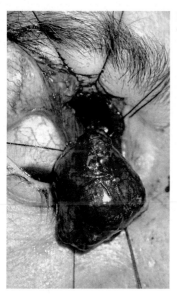

Fig. 11.10 Medial cavernous hemangioma excision via a medial lid split orbitotomy.

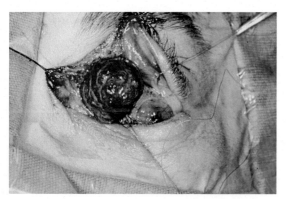

Fig. 11.11 Cavernous hemangioma excision via a lateral orbitotomy.

Lymphangioma

Key Facts

- Benign, diffusely infiltrating vascular orbital or periocular malformation
- Typically identified during first decade, may be present at birth
- **Unknown cause:**
  - arise from pluripotent mesodermal stem cells capable of forming vascular or lymphatic structures
- Uncommon
- Associated lesions may be present in face, oropharynx, or throat
- Difficult to treat

Clinical Findings

- **Presentation in childhood as:**
  - slowly progressive proptosis
  - sudden onset of proptosis due to hemorrhage (chocolate cyst)
  - deep red or bluish, soft, elevated, multilobed lesions of conjunctiva and eyelid
  - a combination of above
- May enlarge after upper respiratory tract infection
- No change with Valsalva maneuver
- Consists of multiple thin-walled, endothelial-lined vascular channels containing lymphocytic aggregations, serous fluid, and blood products

Imaging

- Important in diagnosis
- CT shows multiple contiguous, dilated cystic spaces with varying densities
- Cystic spaces rarely enhance because of no direct connection with circulation
- Extension into central nervous system common

Differential Diagnosis

- Capillary hemangioma, varix, arterial–venous malformation
- Mixed venous anomalies may exist in which combinations of tissues occur together

Treatment

- **Medical:**
  - difficult to manage
  - observation for small lesions
  - corticosteroids and radiotherapy not effective
- **Surgical:**
  - careful surgical debulking to improve deformity
  - cyst drainage when vision threatened after rapid growth or hemorrhage
  - complete resection rarely possible because of infiltrative nature; multiple procedures often required

Prognosis

- Guarded
  - Can be associated with progressive deformity without reasonable options for treatment
- **Possibility of vision loss to:**
  - amblyopia • proptosis • corneal exposure • optic nerve compression

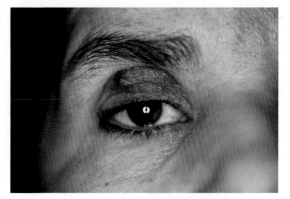

Fig. 11.12 Lesion visible through the right upper eyelid.

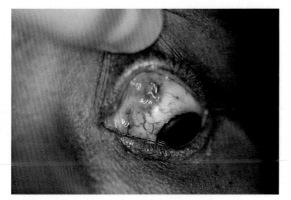

Fig. 11.13 Lymphangioma of the anterior right orbit.

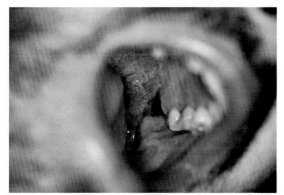

Fig. 11.14 Lesion of the oropharynx.

Optic Nerve Glioma

Key Facts

- Benign tumor of optic nerve, causing optic nerve enlargement
  - Also called juvenile pilocytic astrocytoma
  - Gliomas can occur at other sites along visual pathway
- Uncommon
- About 50% of glioma patients have neurofibromatosis (NF) type 1

Clinical Findings

- Optic nerve tumor seen in childhood
  - 75% diagnosed by age 10
- Solitary fusiform enlargement of optic nerve (Fig. 11.15)
  - Patients present with gradual, painless axial proptosis (Fig. 11.16)
- Visual acuity can be normal but gradually decreases with time
- Early, papilledema may be seen
  - Later, optic atrophy may occur
- Classic radiologic finding is a kink in the anterior portion of the nerve (Fig. 11.17)
- MRI of the tumor is isointense on T_1- and hyperintense on T_2-weighted studies (Fig. 11.18)
- Early diagnosis important to identify chiasmal involvement
- Elongated pilocytic astrocytes form bulk of tumor
  - Cystic spaces can occur
  - Rosenthal fibers (eosinophilic substance in astrocyte) are seen
  - Extension into meninges can cause confusion with meningioma diagnosis

Ancillary Testing

- CT or MRI provides excellent view of orbital portion of tumor
  - Optic nerve calcification does not occur
  - MRI preferred to evaluate posterior extent of tumor

Differential Diagnosis

- Optic nerve meningioma
- Diagnosis of NF type 1 should be considered
  - Bilateral optic nerve tumors are diagnostic of NF

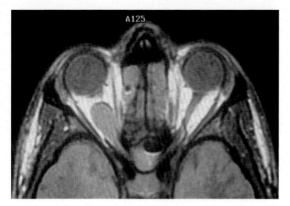

Fig. 11.15 Axial T$_1$-weighted MRI showing isointense fusiform enlargement of the right optic nerve. This tumor extends into the orbital apex.

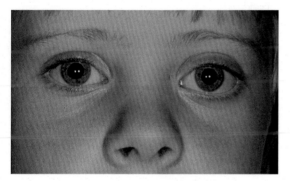

Fig. 11.16 A 4-year-old girl with painless progressive proptosis of the left eye. Note that there is slight downward displacement of the left globe.

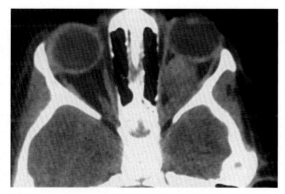

Fig. 11.17 Axial T$_1$-weighted MRI showing the typical kink in the optic nerve seen in this tumor secondary to the mass effect from the tumor.

Treatment

- Based on location of tumor and current vision of patient
- Most cases are observed, with repeated ophthalmic examinations to monitor vision, proptosis, and corneal status every 6–12 months
- Serial MRI studies to monitor for posterior growth of tumor (rarely, if ever, seen)
- Surgical resection for tumors that extend into optic canal, threatening extension into chiasm
  - Blind eyes that present with cosmetically significant proptosis or corneal damage may benefit from tumor removal
  - Transcranial approach to orbit preferred
  - Optic nerve should be resected from chiasm to globe
- Radiation for unresectable optic nerve tumors or when tumor involves chiasm or optic radiations
- Chemotherapy avoids potential radiation effects on bony growth orbit

Prognosis

- Good for tumors confined to orbit
- Intracranial extension can be complicated by involvement of hypothalamus or pituitary gland, which may be associated with endocrine abnormalities or obstructive hydrocephalus

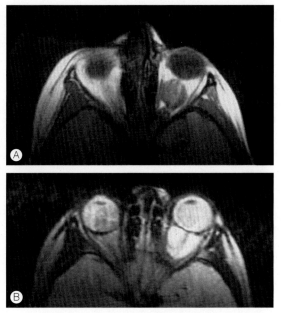

Fig. 11.18 (**A**) The optic nerve glioma is isointense on this T_1-weighted study. (**B**) T_2-weighted MRI with a hyperintense signal from the optic nerve glioma.

Neurofibroma

Key Facts

- Benign peripheral nerve sheath tumor, a hamartoma
- Can arise from cranial nerves to extraocular muscles, sympathetic and parasympathetic fibers, or sensory branches
- Seen as solitary or multiple skin masses
  - Multiple lesions common in neurofibromatosis (NF)
- S-shaped ptosis due to plexiform neurofibroma

Clinical Findings

- Solitary neurofibromas occur in middle age and later
  - These lesions may be superficial or subcutaneous
  - Superficial lesions may be elevated, sometimes pedunculated
  - Deep lesions may be tender or painful
- **Plexiform neuromas:**
  - S-shaped ptosis of upper eyelid caused by plexiform (bag of worms) neurofibroma (Fig. 11.19)
- Proptosis or diplopia for orbital neurofibroma (Fig. 11.20)
- Two types of NF, both autosomal dominant
  - NF type 1: 85% of cases; skin manifestations common (including café-au-lait spots and multiple neurofibromas); also plexiform neuromas, optic nerve glioma, Lisch nodules, sphenoid wing dysplasia (pulsatile exophthalmos)
  - NF type 2: bilateral acoustic neuromas, multiple meningiomas, and other lesions in brain and spinal cord

Ancillary Testing

- CT or MRI for evaluation of orbital plexiform or solitary neurofibroma
- MRI to evaluate optic nerve and central nervous system

Differential Diagnosis

- Rule out systemic disease (NF)

Treatment

- Excision if solitary cutaneous or orbital lesion
- Plexiform neurofibromas are infiltrative, often cannot be completely excised

Prognosis

- Good prognosis for solitary lesions
- Recurrence rate high with plexiform neurofibroma
- Facial nerve palsy with corneal exposure may occur after acoustic neuroma removal. Also check corneal sensation

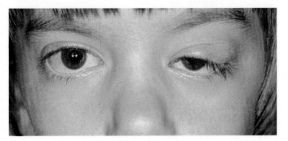

Fig. 11.19 Neurofibroma infiltration of the left upper eyelid. Note the S-shaped configuration of the eyelid.

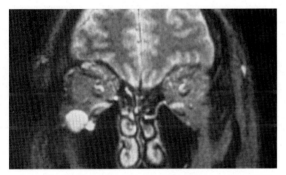

Fig. 11.20 MRI showing enhancing lesion in the right inferior orbit, representing a neurofibroma. This orbital lesion was causing proptosis and diplopia.

Optic Nerve Meningioma

Key Facts

- Benign tumor of optic nerve meninges
- Occurs most commonly in women in third to fourth decades
- Vision loss occurs from growth of tumor within meninges compressing the optic nerve

Clinical Findings

- Gradual unilateral visual loss over years
- Relative afferent pupillary defect on affected side
- Slow, painless, progressive proptosis, but proptosis is usually a late sign (Fig. 11.21)
- Optic nerve head may be normal, swollen, or atrophic
  - Collateral vessels (optociliary) may be present
- Bilateral optic nerve meningiomas (rare) associated with neurofibromatosis type 1
- Tumor contains whorls, or clusters, of meningothelial cells that fill the subarachnoid space and can compress the nerve
  - Psammoma bodies (responsible for calcification on CT scan) may be present
  - Tumor can extend through the dura.

Ancillary Testing

- **CT:**
  - optic nerve enlargement, either localized or fusiform
  - classic railroad track sign may be present, caused by calcification of the tumor in the subarachnoid space (diagnostic, but occurs in a minority of cases) (Fig. 11.22)
- **MRI:**
  - to determine posterior extent of tumor
  - T_1 isointense, T_2 bright, enhances with gadolinium (Fig. 11.23)

Differential Diagnosis

- Optic nerve glioma if tumor present in fusiform pattern
  - Glioma more common in children
- Rarely, other optic nerve infiltrations; sarcoidosis or lymphoma

Treatment

- Observation if the tumor is anterior and vision is good, serial examinations and scans
- Radiation if vision worsens to 20/60, with hope of slowing growth
- Surgical excision if shows posterior extension into optic canal prechiasmal region
  - Transcranial approach resecting tumor from chiasm to globe
- "Stripping" tumor from optic nerve incompletely removes tumor and leaves the eye blind by devascularizing the nerve

Prognosis

- Preservation of vision over long periods because of the slow growth of tumor
- Radiation has been shown to slow tumor growth and vision loss
- Surgical treatment results in blindness and should be reserved for cases with poor vision or intracranial extension

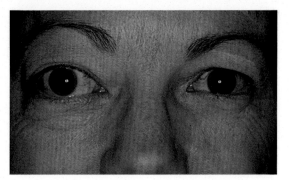

Fig. 11.21 A 57-year-old woman presents with progressive visual loss with axial proptosis of the right eye. Extropia is present.

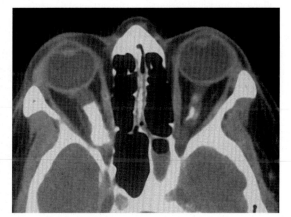

Fig. 11.22 Axial CT showing calcification of right optic nerve meningioma.

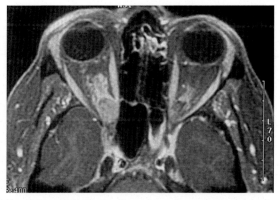

Fig. 11.23 Axial MRI showing right optic nerve enlargement that enhances with gadolinium. The meningioma does not extend into the intracranial space.

Sphenoid Wing Meningioma

Key Facts

- Benign neoplasm arising from meninges
- **Secondary orbital tumor entering orbit through:**
  - superior orbital fissure
  - inferior orbital fissure
  - optic canal
- Apical compression can damage vision
- On imaging, hyperostosis of sphenoid wing is characteristic

Clinical Findings

- Slowly progressive proptosis from bone thickening or orbital extension of tumor
- Fullness of temple from tumor expansion of sphenoid wing
- Normal vision but can experience optic nerve compression with gradual visual loss and visual field changes
- Diplopia possible with orbital invasion or restriction of lateral rectus muscle (Fig. 11.24)

Ancillary Testing

- CT shows bony changes in sphenoid wing (hyperostosis)
  - Tumor extension into orbit can be seen also (Figs 11.24–11.26)
- MRI shows enhancement of tumor with gadolinium
  - Useful to determine intracranial extent of tumor, especially along the dura that appears as a tail from the main tumor
- Visual field changes can occur without visual acuity loss, from slow progressive optic nerve compression

Differential Diagnosis

- Osteoma
- Fibrous dysplasia
- Ossifying fibroma

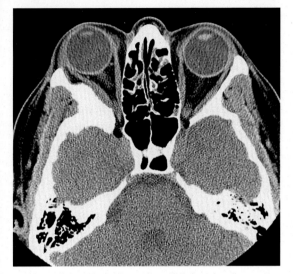

Fig. 11.24 A 35-year-old woman with left periocular swelling. Axial CT shows hyperostosis of the right sphenoid bone. Note the lateral rectus being pushed medially.

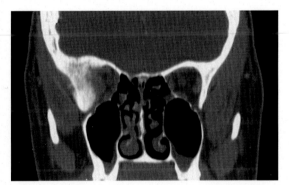

Fig. 11.25 Coronal CT bone window shows a thickened sphenoid bone. The tumor is decreasing the size of the posterior orbit. Optic nerve compression is possible.

Treatment

- Observation appropriate for patients with small non-progressive tumors
- If vision is affected or growth documented, transcranial resection of the tumor, usually including optic canal decompression, is recommended
  - Tumor removal is usually incomplete, because preservation of the function of cranial nerve function is a priority (Fig. 11.26)
- Reconstruction of large orbital roof defects will prevent pulsating exophthalmos
- Radiation therapy after debulking decreases recurrence rate
- Radiation therapy alone may be suitable for elderly patients
- Hormone therapy or chemotherapy generally not useful

Prognosis

- Recurrence of complex incompletely removed tumors occurs over decades
- More localized tumors may be cured
- Risk of malignant transformation extremely small

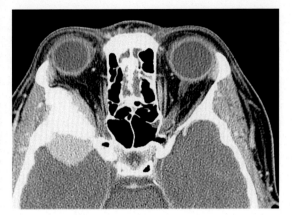

Fig. 11.26 Axial CT with contrast, showing intracranial extension of the meningioma.

Rhabdomyosarcoma

Key Facts

- Most common primary orbital malignancy in children
- Primitive soft tissue tumor of mesenchymal origin
- Rhabdomyosarcoma can occur anywhere in body, but in children occurs most commonly in head and neck
- Although uncommon, diagnosis should be considered in any child with rapidly progressive proptosis

Clinical Findings

- Progressive proptosis in a child, occurring over days to weeks
- Average age is 7.5 years but can occur from birth to late in life
- Diagnosis usually delayed several weeks after onset of signs, with parents attributing the proptosis to minor trauma
- Proptosis can be axial or non-axial depending on position and size of tumor (Figs 11.27 and 11.28)
  - Superonasal quadrant is most common location for the tumor
- Inflammatory signs usually absent

Ancillary Testing

- CT of orbit to characterize tumor
- MRI useful to visualize tumor originating outside but extending into orbit (secondary orbital tumor)
- Imaging may show well-demarcated mass isolated to orbit or destructive lesion extending into orbit (Fig. 11.27B)

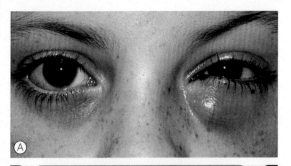

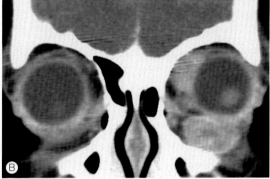

Fig. 11.27 Orbital rhabdomyosarcoma. (**A**) Proptosis and upward displacement of the globe due to inferior mass. (**B**) Coronal CT scan showing well-circumscribed inferior orbital mass without bone erosion.

Rhabdomyosarcoma (Continued)

- **Incisional biopsy (Fig. 11.28B):**
  - send specimens for routine histopathology and immunochemical stains
  - cross-striations (muscle differentiation) are seen in less than half of tumors
- Additional tissue may be sent for electron microscopy or genetic studies (possible mutation in p53 tumor suppressor gene on chromosome 17p13)
- **Four histologic subtypes:**
  1. embryonal (most common)
  2. alveolar (worst prognosis)
  3. pleomorphic (rare in orbit)
  4. botryoid (only in conjunctiva)
- Neck node palpation
  - CT and MRI of head and neck
- Systemic work-up to rule out metastatic disease

Differential Diagnosis

- Bacterial orbital cellulitis
- Lymphangioma
- **Metastatic tumor:**
  - neuroblastoma
  - Ewing sarcoma
- Idiopathic orbital inflammatory disease

Treatment

- Biopsy for diagnosis and staging
- Chemotherapy and radiation (4000–4500 cGy)
- **Complications of chemotherapy:**
  - bone marrow suppression
  - cardiac toxicity
  - respiratory distress
  - metabolic abnormalities
  - secondary malignancies
- **Complications of radiation therapy:**
  - bone growth retardation
  - dermatitis
  - radiation retinopathy
  - enophthalmos
  - dry eye
  - decreased vision

Prognosis

- 5-year survival rate for isolated orbital rhabdomyosarcoma is 95%
  - Orbital exenteration or other extensive surgery not indicated unless conventional therapy fails

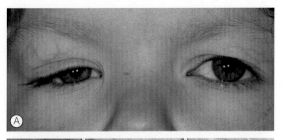

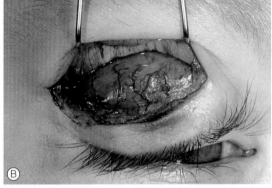

Fig. 11.28 (**A**) Proptosis and ptosis due to superior and retrobulbar mass. (**B**) Anterior orbitotomy for incisional biopsy.

Lymphoproliferative Disorders

Key Facts

- A group of neoplasms arising from lymphoid tissue falling into a spectrum of benign (reactive lymphoid hyperplasia) to malignant (lymphoma) tumors
- Lymphoid tumors represent as much as 20% of orbital mass lesions
- Most periocular lymphoid tumors occur in orbit, most often in lacrimal glands (Fig. 11.29)
  - Unlike other orbital tumors, bilateral lesions are not uncommon
- Biology of the tumor can be categorized based on clinical, histologic, immunohistochemical, and molecular characteristics
  - Based on surface cell markers, three out of four orbital lymphoid lesions are considered malignant lymphomas (90% based on molecular genetic analysis)
- Systemic involvement may or may not be present at time of periocular presentation
- Incidence of subsequent systemic involvement increases over time
  - Orbital lesions considered "benign" pathologically may show eventual systemic involvement

Clinical Findings

- Periocular lymphoid lesions can be seen in conjunctiva, orbit, or eyelids
  - Lacrimal gland enlargement is most common, but a lymphoid mass may appear anywhere in the orbit
- Most present as a progressively enlarging painless mass, usually anterior
- Conjunctival lymphoma tends to be isolated and not systemic at time of diagnosis (Fig. 11.30)
- Systemic disease may have been previously diagnosed, occur concomitantly, or occur in the future
- Most common lymphoma is mucosa-associated lymphoid tissue (MALT) type, also known as marginal zone lymphoma

Ancillary Testing

- Orbital imaging with CT or MRI
  - Typically lymphoid mass "molds" to shape of the globe
  - Does not erode bone

Differential Diagnosis

- **Other causes of lacrimal gland enlargement:**
  - lacrimal gland infiltrations such as sarcoidosis
  - primary lacrimal gland tumor such as benign mixed tumor
- Other orbital mass lesions

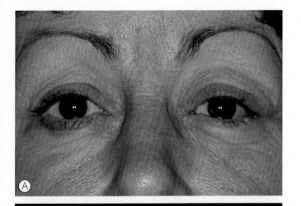

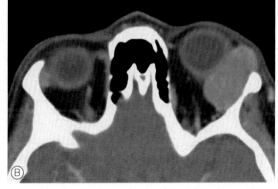

Fig. 11.29 Orbital lymphoma. (**A**) Subtle ptosis, minimal proptosis, and a palpable anterior mass in the upper left eyelid. (**B**) CT scan showing an enlarged lacrimal gland. Note smooth shape "pushing" into the orbit without any change in the surrounding bone.

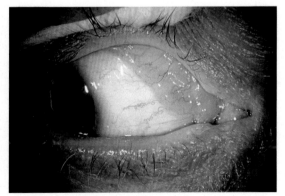

Fig. 11.30 Conjunctival lymphoma: salmon patch.

Lymphoproliferative Disorders (Continued)

Treatment

- Incisional biopsy for diagnosis, fixed and fresh tissue (Fig. 11.31)
- **Refer to oncology for systemic evaluation:**
  - H&P
  - chest and abdominal CT
  - bone marrow
- Radiation therapy for isolated periocular lesion
- Chemotherapy for systemic disease

Prognosis

- Visual function usually not affected
- MALT-type tumors tend to occur elsewhere slowly over years, with as many as 50% becoming systemic over 10 years
  - Higher grade lymphomas may be fatal within months

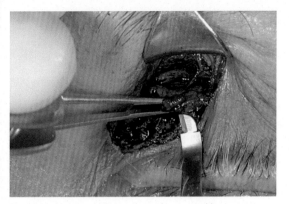
Fig. 11.31 Incisional biopsy through upper skin crease: anterior orbital mass proven to be lymphoma.

Benign Mixed Tumor of the Lacrimal Gland

Key Facts

- Rare primary epithelial neoplasm of lacrimal gland
- 50% of all epithelial lacrimal gland tumors are benign mixed tumors (pleomorphic adenomas)
- Histopathology shows proliferation of both epithelial and mesenchymal elements
- 25% of all lacrimal fossa masses, 3% of orbital tumors
- Surgical excision with intact pseudocapsule is a cure in most patients

Clinical Findings

- Slowly progressive (>1 year), painless proptosis, inferior-medial globe displacement, and upper eyelid swelling
- Most commonly seen in 20- to 50-year-old patients
- Non-tender, firm mass, sometimes palpable at superior-temporal rim
- Histopathology shows mixed involvement of both epithelial and mesenchymal elements

Imaging

- **CT of orbit:**
  - round or oval, well-circumscribed mass in superior-temporal orbit
  - bone remodeling or "fossa" formation adjacent to lacrimal gland very common
  - no evidence of bone erosion or destruction (suggests malignancy)
- MRI not necessary

Differential Diagnosis

- Malignant epithelial tumors of lacrimal gland
  - A unilateral lacrimal gland mass that presents with similar signs but present <1 year or associated pain and numbness suggests malignancy, usually adenoid cystic carcinoma of lacrimal gland
- **Lacrimal gland infiltrations:**
  - lymphoid tumors • inflammatory and infectious lesions

Treatment

- No medical treatment
  - Observation is not appropriate
- Complete en bloc surgical excision of tumor and intact pseudocapsule via lateral orbitotomy for lesions clinically and radiographically consistent with benign mixed tumor
- Preliminary frozen section testing before complete excision may be appropriate for atypical presentations (most often lymphoid infiltration)
  - Preferable not to violate the capsule and remove any suspicious lesion in its entirety

Prognosis

- Malignant degeneration reported in up to 32% of cases with incomplete excision
- Low recurrence rate when excision performed with intact pseudocapsule
- Late recurrences possible, so long-term follow-up indicated
- Late recurrence may indicate malignant degeneration in as much as 10% at 20 years' and 20% at 30 years' follow-up (malignant mixed tumor)

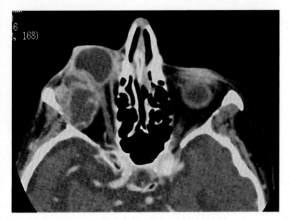

Fig. 11.32 CT scan showing a large right orbital pleomorphic adenoma. Note the globe indentation.

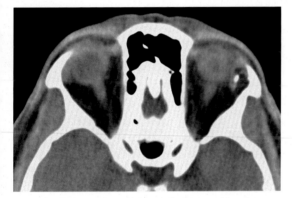

Fig. 11.33 CT scan showing a small pleomorphic adenoma of the left orbit. While not typical, note the cystic area of the tumor with some calcification of the cyst wall.

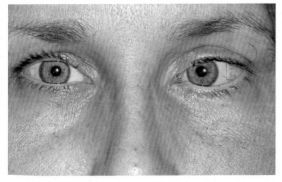

Fig. 11.34 Left-sided proptosis and medial globe displacement in a patient with a benign lacrimal gland mass.

Adenoid Cystic Carcinoma of the Lacrimal Gland

Key Facts

- Most common primary epithelial malignancy of lacrimal gland
- Rare tumor
- Occurs most commonly in fourth decade
- Symptoms for <1 year, pain, and bony erosion on CT are typical of malignant lacrimal gland lesions
- Local intracranial spread and perineural invasion leads to a very poor prognosis

Clinical Findings

- Progressive proptosis and globe displacement, eyelid swelling, and motility disturbances are common
- Pain is a common finding (70%)
- Numbness (trigeminal nerve distribution), decreased visual acuity, and choroidal folds may be present
- Palpable mass may be present in superior-temporal orbit

Imaging

- **CT:**
  - enlarged infiltrative lacrimal gland mass
  - bony erosion typical
  - calcification common
  - extension into superior orbital fissure possible
- MRI for any suspected intracranial spread

Pathology

- Non-encapsulated mass with aggressive malignant glandular cells often invading neurons
- Classic cribiform Swiss cheese pattern most common

Differential Diagnosis

- Malignant mixed cell, primary adenocarcinoma, mucoepidermoid carcinomas
- Benign mixed tumor
- Other infiltrative lacrimal gland conditions

Treatment

- Controversial—no evidence that any treatment prolongs survival
- Complete surgical excision (en bloc, exenteration, extended exenteration with craniofacial resection) usually offered
- Usually radiotherapy after surgical excision

Prognosis

- Poor
- Local recurrences and cranial invasion typical
  - Perineural spread difficult to treat
- Metastatic spread, especially to lung, common, may occur years after primary excision

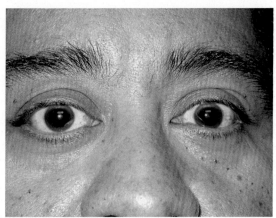

Fig. 11.35 A 48-year-old patient with a 2-month history of proptosis and pain. Note downward displacement of right globe.

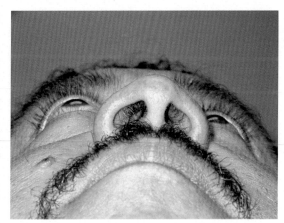

Fig. 11.36 The same patient as in Fig. 11.35. "Worm's" eye view.

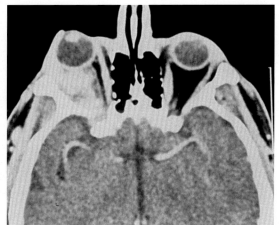

Fig. 11.37 CT showing a diffusely infiltrative adenoid cystic carcinoma of the right orbit.

Pediatric Metastatic Orbital Disease

Key Facts

- **Most orbital tumors in children are not malignancies, but developmental:**
  - hamartomas • choristomas (hemangiomas, lymphangiomas, dermoid cysts)
- Most common orbital metastases in children include neuroblastoma and masses arising from cellular collections due to leukemia
- The most common primary tumor is rhabdomyosarcoma (see *Rhabdomyosarcoma*)
- Metastatic orbital disease is rare
  - Metastatic disease in children more commonly appears in the orbit than in the choroid
- A history of previous cancer is important
- **Diagnosis made by:**
  - clinical examination
  - imaging
  - biopsy
- Treatment is usually coordinated by a pediatric oncologist, often with radiation oncology consultation
- The orbital presentation may be the initial sign of unrealized primary tumor
- Even if the patient reports that the cancer is in remission, metastatic disease must be ruled out

Metastatic Neuroblastoma

- Neoplasm arising from undifferentiated neural crest cells, usually originating in neck, abdomen, or mediastinum
- Second to rhabdomyosarcoma in frequency of orbital tumors in children
- Proptosis and periocular ecchymosis from hemorrhagic necrosis of tumor is common presentation
- Orbital metastasis frequently occurs (Figs 11.38 and 11.39)
- Horner syndrome possible if sympathetic chain involved with tumor

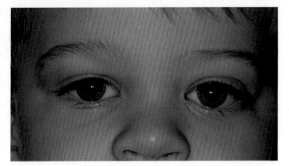

Fig. 11.38 A 4-year-old with fullness in the left upper eyelid and left inferior globe displacement.

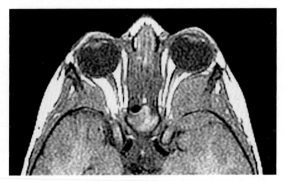

Fig. 11.39 MRI shows bilateral lateral orbital masses, the larger mass on the left. Both masses are isointense on T_1. The left mass has intracranial extension.

- CT shows soft tissue mass (Fig. 11.40)
  - Lateral orbital wall bone involvement with destructive lesions common
- **Urine test for elevated:**
  - homovanillic acid
  - vanillylmandelic acid
  - 3-methoxy-4-hydroxyphenylethyleneglycol
- Treatment is chemotherapy and orbital radiation
- Guarded prognosis for survival

Orbital Involvement with Leukemia

- Orbital manifestation of a systemic malignancy, usually appearing in late stages of leukemia
- May present with axial proptosis or other globe displacement, may be bilateral
- Occurs in acute lymphoblastic leukemia most commonly
  - Can be seen in myelogenous leukemia; the orbital infiltrate is known as a granulocytic sarcoma or chloroma
- CT or MRI used to characterize the lesion (Fig. 11.41)
- Incisional biopsy
  - Histopathology: Leder stain confirms presence of esterase and lysosomal enzymes that are seen in granulocytic process
- Chemotherapy for systemic disorder
  - Survival is better if orbital lesion identified before advanced systemic disease occurs
- Prognosis improved with current chemotherapeutic regimens

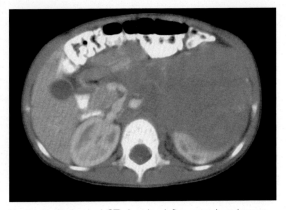

Fig. 11.40 Abdominal CT showing left supraadrenal mass with calcification.

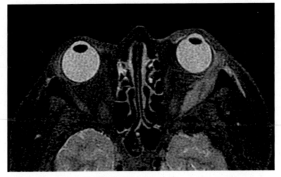

Fig. 11.41 MRI T$_2$-weighted image showing infiltrative mass in the right lateral orbit including the lateral rectus muscle in a patient with myelogenous leukemia.

Metastatic Orbital Disease in Adults

Key Facts

- Metastatic orbital disease is rare, 2–10% of orbital tumors
- In adults, metastases appear more commonly in the choroid than in the orbit
- **Most common primary tumors:**
  - lung
  - breast
  - prostate
- Lymphoid tumors in adults are not considered metastatic lesions, rather as manifestations of a systemic malignancy
- **Common presentations include:**
  - proptosis
  - diplopia
  - palpable mass
  - orbital discomfort
- Rapidly growing metastases may cause pain and signs of inflammation due to tissue or bone destruction
- 75% of patients have a known primary tumor
  - Even if the patient reports that the cancer is in remission, you must rule out metastatic disease
- **Diagnosis made by:**
  - clinical examination
  - imaging
  - biopsy
- Treatment usually coordinated by oncologist, often with radiation oncology consultation
- Orbital presentation may be initial sign of unrealized primary tumor

Metastatic Breast Cancer

- Most common metastatic lesion in women
- Most often presents as infiltrative lesion that affects extraocular muscles, leading to restrictive deficit (Fig. 11.42)
- Like most adult metastatic disease, choroidal metastasis is more common than orbital metastasis (Fig. 11.43)
- Breast cancer is classic cause of enophthalmos in a patient with an orbital mass—caused by the tissue contraction that occurs with scirrhous adenocarcinoma
- May cause exophthalmos in some cases

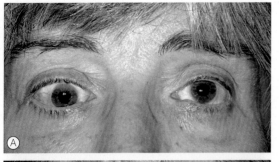

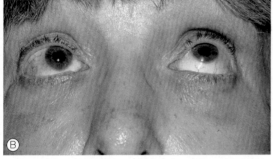

Fig. 11.42 (A) A 57-year-old woman with gradual onset of diplopia. Right hypotropia in primary gaze. (B) Limited motility in upgaze of the right eye.

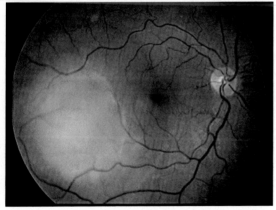

Fig. 11.43 Whitish choroidal mass in the temporal retina of the right eye. There is subretinal fluid around the mass.

- Usually imaged by CT but can use MRI (Fig. 11.44)
  - Extraocular muscle or soft tissue infiltration, or bony destruction
  - MRI findings are a hypointense mass on T_1-weighted images and hyperintense signals on T_2-weighted or contrast studies
- Differential diagnosis
  Differential diagnosis includes thyroid eye disease
  - Both are common in women and can have a restrictive ocular motility defect
  Incisional biopsy is performed if known metastatic disease does not exist
  - Work-up includes hormone receptor studies and systemic oncology evaluation
- Treatment
  Treatment options include:
  - hormone therapy (tamoxifen)
  - chemotherapy or radiation to orbit
- Prognosis
  Metastatic disease often occurs many years after initial diagnosis
  - Onset of metastatic disease in one location often suggests widespread disease

Bronchogenic Carcinoma

- Seen in middle-aged to older patients
- Time interval between diagnosis of primary disease and metastasis is months
- Metastasizes to the choroid more frequent than to the orbit
- Proptosis from tumor mass effect
  - Motility deficits, pain, and chemosis are frequent (Fig. 11.45)
- CT and MRI usually show an infiltrative mass
  - Bone destruction is common
- Incisional biopsy is performed, then systemic work-up by oncologist
- **Palliation is the rule:**
  - orbital radiation in most cases, chemotherapy in some cases
- Metastatic disease has a poor prognosis
  - Survival is usually <1 year

Prostate Carcinoma

- Proptosis, diplopia, and ptosis most common presenting signs (Fig. 11.46)
- Equal or second to lung as primary site in men
  - CT and MRI—most common orbital site is bone, with osteoclastic and osteoblastic response (Fig. 11.47)
  - Uncommonly can present as a solitary lesion of extraocular muscle mass (Fig. 11.48)
- **Serology:**
  - prostate specific antigen levels
- Other metastatic sites include spine and long bones
- Incisional biopsy, especially if no other metastatic disease is known
- Oncologist evaluation
- **Treatment:**
  - orbital radiation in most patients
  - hormonal therapy or other chemotherapy for systemic spread
- Patients usually live a long time after metastases first diagnosed

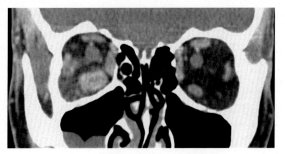

Fig. 11.44 Coronal CT showing an enlarged right inferior rectus muscle from metastatic breast disease.

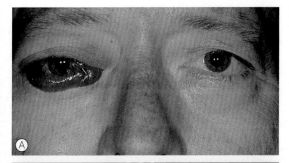

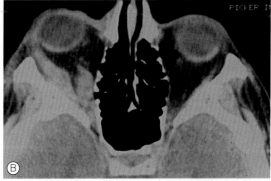

Fig. 11.45 (**A**) Marked chemosis in this 68-year-old man with known bronchogenic carcinoma. (**B**) Axial CT showing the metastasis involving the right lateral rectus muscle and proptosis of the eye.

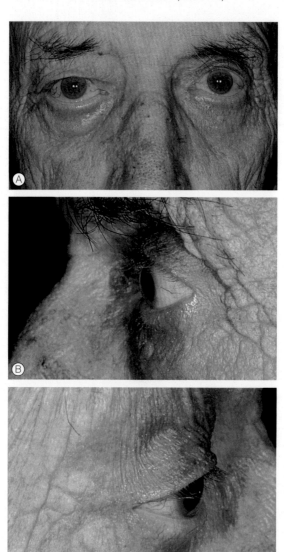

Fig. 11.46 (**A**) A 68-year-old male presented with globe ptosis and proptosis. (**B**) Profile view of the left eye in normal position (**C**) Profile view showing marked proptosis of the right eye.

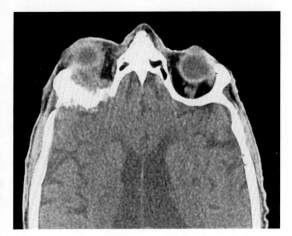

Fig. 11.47 Axial CT showing osteoblastic changes along the lateral wall and sphenoid bone in the right orbit. This bony change was the result of metastatic prostate carcinoma.

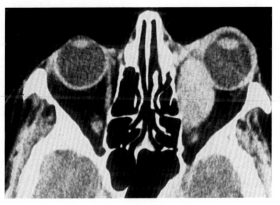

Fig. 11.48 Diffuse enlargement of the right medial rectus muscle from recurrent metastatic prostate process. The muscle was biopsied for confirmation of metastatic disease in a patient previously in remission.

Section
12
Disorders of the Orbit: Vascular Abnormalities

Arteriovenous Fistula

Key Facts

- Abnormal direct connection between arterial and venous circulations, without an intervening capillary net
- Ocular signs due to rupture of internal carotid or smaller branches of carotid system into cavernous sinus, leading to reversed flow of venous system supplying the eye
- **Two types of carotid cavernous sinus fistulas:**
  1. high flow, with branches of the carotid flowing into the cavernous sinus
  2. low flow, caused by dural arteries flowing into cavernous sinus; sometimes also called indirect fistulas, because the miscommunication is not directly from the carotid artery but from its meningeal branches
- Traumatic cause in 70–90% of high-flow carotid-sinus fistulas
- Spontaneous etiology more common in low-flow dural-sinus fistulas
- Uncommon
- Spontaneous low-flow fistulas more common in females than in males

Clinical Findings

- Decreased visual acuity in 50–75%
- **Orbital congestion:**
  - dilated conjunctival corkscrew vessels, chemosis
  - proptosis (may be pulsatile if flow is high)
  - increased IOP
  - central retinal artery or vein occlusion
- Corneal exposure
- Cranial neuropathy including 3, 6, and 7

Imaging

- Cerebral angiogram is the gold standard
- **CT or MRI show:**
  - dilated superior ophthalmic vein • enlarged extraocular muscles • fullness of cavernous sinus

Differential Diagnosis

- Orbital vascular tumors, inflammations, orbital infection

Treatment

- **Medical therapy:**
  - antiglaucoma medications for increased IOP
  - many (20–50%) dural fistulas close spontaneously
  - lubricants to protect the cornea
- **Surgical:**
  - endovascular closure using balloons, wires, or coils via direct carotid or transvenous (superior ophthalmic vein) approach
- **Complications:**
  - cerebral angiogram and interventional radiologic procedures are associated with risks, including stroke and death

Prognosis

- Treatment is effective at reversing all signs and symptoms
  - Vision loss usually improves

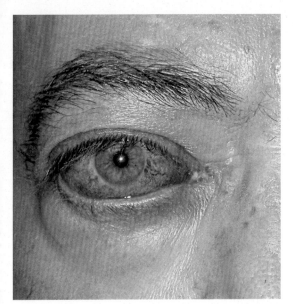

Fig. 12.1 A right-sided low-flow (dural-sinus) fistula after a motor vehicle accident. It closed spontaneously 6 weeks after the trauma.

Orbital Varix

Key Facts

- A congenital venous malformation
- Dilatation of involved veins presumably is due to venous wall weakness
- May cause pain and proptosis due to orbital hemorrhage or thrombosis
- Generally no treatment is usually required

Clinical Findings

- Pressure sensation with any activity that increases venous pressure, such as Valsalva maneuver or dependent head position
- Examination may be normal
- Proptosis that varies with Valsalva may be seen
- In unusual cases, varix may extend anteriorly and be visible

Ancillary Testing

- **CT or MRI of orbits with contrast:**
  - Valsalva maneuver during scan or
  - head in dependent position

Differential Diagnosis

- Generally, other vascular lesions of the orbit (e.g. cavernous hemangioma or hemangiopericytoma) appear differently as circumscribed masses
  - These lesions do not vary with Valsalva maneuver
- Arteriovenous malformation may have similar imaging characteristics, but clinical examination is different due to arterial nature of flow
  - These lesions will not change in size during Valsalva maneuver, unlike a varix

Treatment

- Observation
- Surgical intervention if bleeding or thrombosis threaten vision
- Hemostasis can be difficult, because vessel caliber can be large and walls thin

Prognosis

- Generally stable over time
  - Very few patients require any intervention
- Most patients can control symptoms by avoiding activities that increase venous pressure

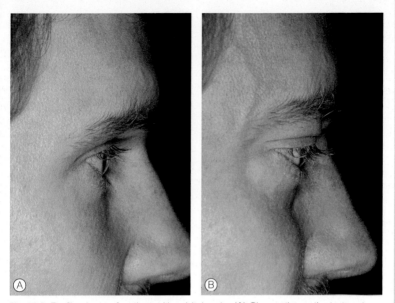

Fig. 12.2 Profile views of patient with orbital varix. (**A**) Shows the patient at rest. (**B**) Shows the patient while performing a valsalva maneuver. Note proptosis of the right eye.

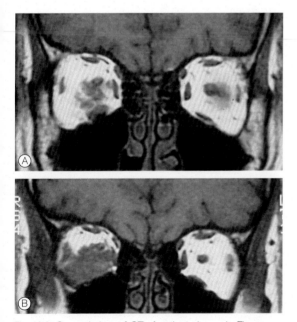

Fig. 12.3 Coronal view of CT of patient shown in Figure 12.2. (**A**) Shows a soft tissue density lesion above the inferior rectus muscle. (**B**) The lesion has now enlarged during a Valsalva maneuver that increased venous pressure and expanded the varix.

Section

13

Disorders of the Orbit: Trauma

Traumatic Optic Neuropathy

Key Facts

- Loss of vision resulting from indirect injury to optic nerve
  - Force of injury transferred through orbital bones to canalicular portion of optic nerve
  - Shearing action on tethered nerve damages microcirculation to nerve, leading to optic nerve edema and death
- Craniomaxillofacial trauma, most commonly to superior-lateral orbital rim, from motor vehicle accidents, assaults, or falls
  - Can result from seemingly insignificant trauma
- Diagnosis easiest if there is no associated ocular injury
- Rare, most common in young males
- An object penetrating orbit or a bone fragment may cause "direct" injury to the nerve. In these cases, the offending object should be removed

Clinical Findings

- Decreased visual acuity
- Visual field defects
- Relative afferent papillary defect
  - May be only sign in an unresponsive patient

Imaging

- CT is study of choice
  - Order thin slice coronal and axial cuts with bone and soft tissue windows
- Orbital fractures commonly associated with traumatic optic neuropathy (TON) (50–85%)
- Optic canal fractures present in ≤40% of cases

Differential Diagnosis

- **Other causes of decreased vision:**
  - "direct" injury • ocular injury • optic nerve avulsion • optic nerve hematoma • orbital hemorrhage • intracranial injury

Treatment

- **Medical:**
  - treatment is controversial and effectiveness of medical and/or surgical therapy unproven • corticosteroids shown to be effective in some studies, often used in doses used in spinal cord injury • methylprednisolone 30 mg/kg loading followed by 5.4 mg/kg per h for 48 h, discontinue if no response, taper slowly if effective, and observe closely for deterioration • Results of CRASH study show that intravenous steroid use is associated with higher mortality in patients with significant head injury; this has prompted many ophthalmologists to not use steroids for TON if associated with other severe head injury
- **Surgical:**
  - canthotomy or cantholysis for increased intraorbital pressure • removal of bony fractures impinging on optic nerve (direct trauma) • optic canal decompression for cases unresponsive to corticosteroids (controversial)

Prognosis

- Guarded in all cases
- Profound visual loss common
- Severity of initial visual loss correlates with worse prognosis for recovery

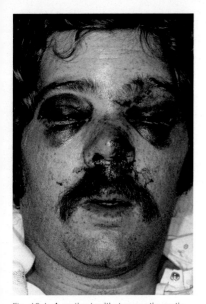

Fig. 13.1 A patient with traumatic optic neuropathy after a motor vehicle accident.

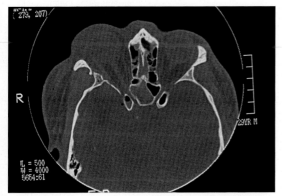

Fig. 13.2 A right optic canal fracture. Note the fracture of the medial optic canal wall (lateral sphenoid sinus wall).

Blowout Fracture

Key Facts

- Most common orbital fracture seen by an ophthalmologist
- Two theories on etiology of this injury
  - Occurs with blunt trauma to face with an object larger than the anterior orbital opening; increased intraorbital pressure causes the thin bones of the orbital floor or medial wall to fracture
  - Blunt force to the inferior orbital rim causes a buckling effort on the floor and leads to fracture
- With either mechanism, a significant amount of orbital tissue may become entrapped at the site, limiting ocular motility (Fig. 13.3), or cause enophthalmos
- Associated with significant ocular injury in ≥10% of cases

Clinical Findings

- Swelling and ecchymosis of the eyelids
- Emphysema of eyelids, implying a fracture into the sinus (Fig. 13.4)
- **Small fractures:**
  - diplopia secondary to inferior rectus or orbital tissue entrapment or muscle paresis (Fig. 13.5)
  - pain with vertical eye movement
- **Large fractures:**
  - enophthalmos occurs due to increased orbital volume
  - exophthalmos may be present at time of injury due to edema or hemorrhage
- Hypesthesia of ipsilateral cheek, side of nose, upper lip, and gums from infraorbital nerve injury
- Medial wall fractures present often with restriction to abduction and adduction with enophthalmos

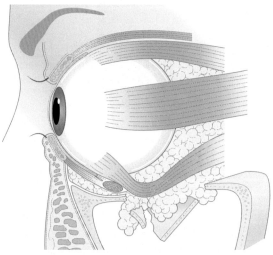

Fig. 13.3 The orbital floor buckling after increased intraorbital pressure. The inferior orbital contents have herniated into the fracture site. This herniation leads to motility disturbance and possible enophthalmos.

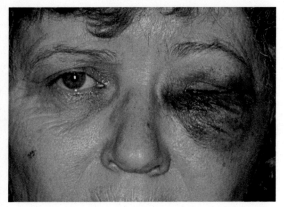

Fig. 13.4 Periocular ecchymosis and emphysema from a blowout fracture. This patient had a coughing episode that led to air in the left orbit and eyelids.

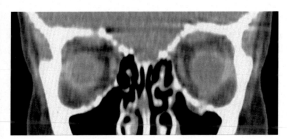

Fig. 13.5 Coronal CT showing a small left orbital floor fracture with tissue entrapment.

- In children, orbital floor fractures can occur with minimal signs of trauma—so-called white-eyed blowout
  - Marked restriction to ocular motility due to trapdoor impingement of orbital tissue
  - Patient may experience bradycardia with vertical eye movement due to the oculocardiac reflex (Fig. 13.6)
  - Urgent repair (24–48 h) required to release pressure on the entrapped tissue before tissue ischemia causes permanent muscle scarring
- Caution any blowout patient about blowing nose or sneezing with the mouth closed
  - These activities can force air from the sinus into the orbit

Ancillary Testing

- **CT:**
  - thin cuts (1.5–2 mm), coronal view shows floor best (Fig. 13.7)
- **Forced ductions:**
  - helpful in determining if the orbital tissues are entrapped in the fracture site

Differential Diagnosis

- Trimalar (zygomaticomalar complex) fracture (common)
- **Silent sinus syndrome causing enophthalmos:**
  - motility normal • no history of trauma • resulting from maxillary sinus disease

Treatment

- **Indications for surgical repair:**
  - diplopia, especially in primary or reading position
  - enophthalmos >2 mm
  - large floor fracture such that enophthalmos is predicted
- In adults, repair within 2 weeks; in childhood white-eyed blowout, repair urgently
- **Operation:**
  - forced duction test (FDT) to show entrapment
  - exposure of orbital fracture through a transconjunctival incision
  - elevate entrapped tissue from fracture site
  - place an implant over the fracture site to prevent tissue from dropping back into fracture site (Fig. 13.8)
  - recheck FDT after placement of implant
  - medial wall fractures can be approached from the floor and through a transcaruncular incision

Prognosis

- Most patients will have functional single vision and no enophthalmos after repair
- White-eyed blowout fractures in children have poor prognosis if not repaired within 24–48 h
- Late onset enophthalmos possibly due to fat atrophy
- **Rare complications of repair:**
  - loss of vision • persistent diplopia • eyelid retraction • enophthalmos

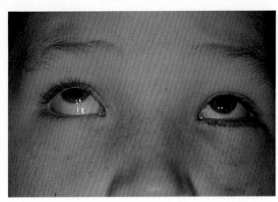

Fig. 13.6 Motility in this 6-year-old boy showed marked restriction to up gaze. There is very little evidence of the blunt trauma that led to the fracture. The injury was repaired the same day of the patient's evaluation.

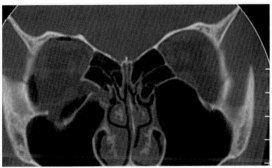

Fig. 13.7 Coronal CT showing a large right orbital floor fracture. The black area in the orbit represents air. The bony fragment is displaced into the maxillary sinus, enlarging the orbital volume. There is no tissue entrapment and the motility was normal.

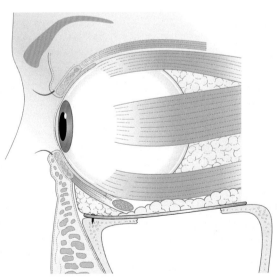

Fig. 13.8 Repair of the floor fracture with an implant placed over the fracture site. The implant is secured to the orbital rim with a small titanium screw and prevents the orbital tissue from falling back into the fracture site.

Zygomaticomaxillary Complex Fracture

Key Facts

- Common facial fracture due to motor vehicle accident or fist injury to cheek
- **Also called a tripod fracture, as fractures are seen in three places:**
  - frontozygomatic suture
  - zygomatic arch
  - inferior orbital rim extending into the zygomatic buttress
- Orbital floor is always fractured
  - Malar complex displacement determines ocular signs

Clinical Findings

- Ecchymosis and edema of eyelids and cheek imply serious injury (Fig. 13.9)
- Subcutaneous emphysema suggests fracture into sinus V2
  - Hypesthesia implies a fracture involving the floor
- **Diagnosis is made by:**
  - flattened malar eminence
  - inferior displacement of lateral canthus
  - palpable step on inferior rim
- Diplopia, enophthalmos, and globe ptosis are associated with significant displacement of malar complex
- Trismus can occur due to swelling or impingement of the arch on the coronoid process of the mandible

Ancillary Testing

- CT scan to evaluate extent of facial fracture (Fig. 13.10)
- **Forced duction testing:**
  - diplopia is usually due to tissue swelling or globe displacement, not restriction

Differential Diagnosis

- Other orbital fractures including blowout or Le Fort fracture

Treatment

- **Exposure:**
  - canthotomy or cantholysis and transconjunctival incision exposes frontozygomatic suture and inferior rim fracture
  - gingivobuccal incision exposes zygomatic buttress
- **Reduction:**
  - three-dimensional alignment of fractured segments
  - views of floor and lateral orbital wall with reduction
- **Rigid internal fixation:**
  - titanium plates to fixate two or more of the fracture lines (zygomatic buttress, inferior orbital rim, and frontozygomatic suture)
- Floor implant if significant disruption of floor persists after aligning fractures

Prognosis

- Accurate reduction restores orbit and cheek anatomy
  - Rigid fixation maintains alignment and stability
- **Complications include:**
  - enophthalmos
  - diplopia
  - facial asymmetry

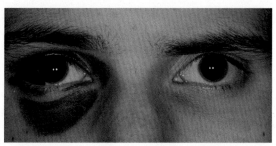

Fig. 13.9 Periocular ecchymosis and subconjunctival hemorrhage after suffering blunt trauma to the right side of the face in a motor vehicle accident. Right malar eminence is slightly flat. There is no globe displacement.

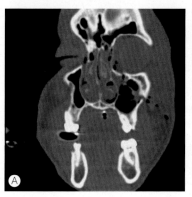 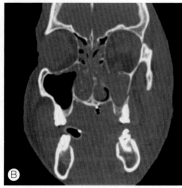

Fig. 13.10 (**A**) Coronal CT showing the left inferior orbital rim fracture. (**B**) Coronal CT midorbit, showing large orbital floor fracture. Note fracture of the zygomatic buttress.

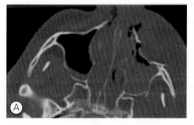 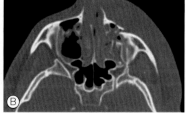

Fig. 13.11 (**A**) Axial CT at the level of the maxillary sinus. The anterior face of the sinus is fractured. (**B**) The fractures extend to the zygomatic buttress.

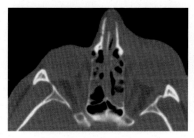

Fig. 13.12 Axial CT showing the fracture of the lateral wall at the zygomaticosphenoid sature.

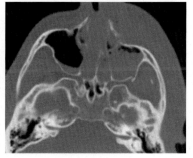

Fig. 13.13 Axial CT of a tripod fracture with an intact zygomatic arch. The arch is not always fractured with a tripod fracture.

LeFort Fracture

Key Facts

- Classification system of midfacial fractures describing which segment of the facial bones are fractured from the normal attachments at the skull base
- Orbital bones are involved in LeFort types II and III (Fig. 13.14)
- Most common after motor vehicle accidents
- Associated eye injuries common

Clinical Findings

- Extreme facial swelling, subcutaneous emphysema, and facial deformity suggest a fracture
- **LeFort type I** fractures separate maxillary teeth from skull
- **LeFort type II** fractures, described as pyramidal fractures, separate the middle portion of the face from the skull, involving the anteromedial portion of the orbit
  - The zygomas remain attached at the frontozygomatic suture
- **LeFort type III** fractures extend more superiorly and posteriorly into the orbit
  - The entire face, including the zygomas, is detached from the skull
  - Bilateral LeFort type III fractures are known as craniofacial dysjunction
- The specific type of LeFort fracture is diagnosed radiologically, not clinically
- LeFort fractures may be unilateral or bilateral, symmetric or asymmetric

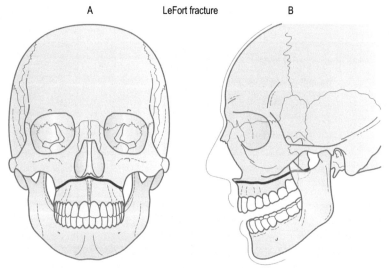

A   LeFort fracture   B

Fig. 13.14 LeFort fracture types. (**A** and **B**) Type I: hard palate is separated from midface, orbits are not involved.

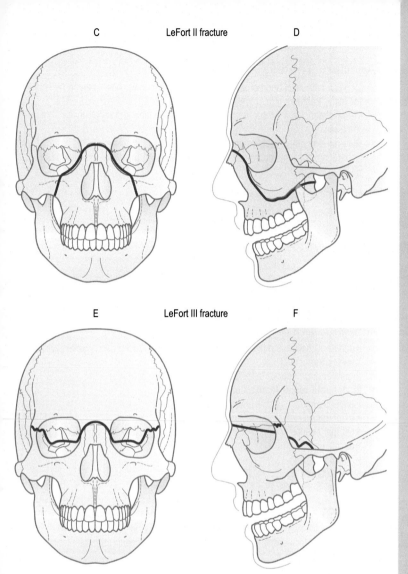

C   LeFort II fracture   D

E   LeFort III fracture   F

Fig. 13.14, cont'd (**C** and **D**) Type II (pyramidal fracture): maxilla is separated from zygomatic complex, anterior orbit is involved. (**E** and **F**) Type III (craniofacial dysjunction): all the facial bones are separated from the skull, fractures occur in the mid and posterior orbit. (From Nerad JA 2001 Oculoplastic Surgery: the Requisites in Ophthalmology. Mosby, St. Louis.)

Ancillary Testing

- CT scan with axial and coronal fine cuts, bone windows, best imaging technique for facial fractures (Fig. 13.15)
- Three-dimensional CT scans are helpful to understand and repair these complex fractures
- Rule out any other multisystem trauma
- Separation from the skull base by fracturing through the pterygoid plates is diagnostic (Fig. 13.15A)

Differential Diagnosis

- Other types of facial fractures

Treatment

- Diagnose and treat any associated eye injuries
- **Exposure:**
  - small periocular, intraoral, and sometime scalp incisions
- **Reduction and fixation:**
  - fractured segments are reduced three-dimensionally and held in position with titanium plates (rigid internal fixation)
  - dental occlusion is used as a guide to maxillary reduction and subsequent facial bone alignment
- Repair of large floor defects requires implant placement
- **Inadequate repair leaves deformities such as:**
  - enophthalmos
  - globe ptosis
  - canthal malposition
  - diplopia
  - malar flattening
  - malocclusion
- Damage to vision is a very rare complication of repair

Prognosis

- Prognosis for normal vision and facial structure is good
- Best chance for normal bone reduction is at the first repair attempt

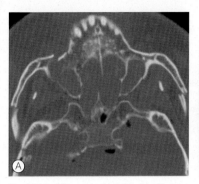
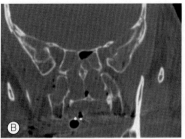

Fig. 13.15 CT scan of bilateral LeFort type III fracture. (**A**) Coronal scan (bone windows) showing fractures through both pterygoid plates. (**B**) There is a right-sided skull fracture and a left-sided optic canal fracture (orbital roof fracture anterior to the canal is seen on this cut).

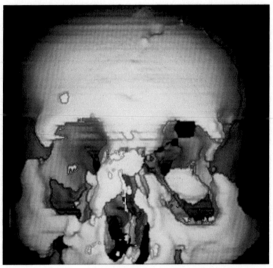

Fig. 13.16 LeFort type III three-dimensional CT scan. The facial bones are separated from the skull (craniofacial dysjunction). (From Nerad JA 2001 Oculoplastic Surgery: the Requisites in Ophthalmology. Mosby, St. Louis.)

Intraorbital Foreign Body

Key Facts

- Suspect with any history of penetrating injury to periocular area • Diagnosis usually made with imaging • All organic foreign bodies should be removed
- Most metallic foreign bodies are well tolerated
  - However, they may be a contraindication for later MRI • Removal, if relatively easy, should be considered

Clinical Findings

- Entrance site may be obvious or not readily visible, sometimes outside the orbital rims (Fig. 13.17) • Rule out ocular injury • Rule out intracranial penetration
- **Try to determine type of foreign body:**
  - glass • metal • vegetable • plastic
- Late onset infection or fistula can occur from retained organic material

Ancillary Testing

- Plain radiographs can be used as a screening test to locate radio-opaque foreign bodies (Fig. 13.18)
- CT or MRI should be obtained if a foreign body is suspected (Fig. 13.19)
  - Organic foreign bodies may not be visible on CT but visible on MRI (Fig. 13.20)
    - Avoid MRI if a metallic foreign body is suspected • If you can ascertain that the metal is non-ferromagnetic, MRI is possible

Differential Diagnosis

- Dried organic foreign bodies may look like air on CT scan • A phlebolith (calcification in a vessel) can be confused with a foreign body

Treatment

- Observation if foreign body is inert (e.g. metallic foreign body), especially if in posterior orbit
- **Indications for surgical removal:**
  - any organic foreign body • a foreign body easily accessible in anterior orbit
    - a foreign body limiting ocular motility or affecting vision
- Weigh potential risk of surgery against risk of complication if leaving foreign body in position

Prognosis

- Most metallic foreign bodies are well tolerated • It is difficult to find small deep orbital foreign bodies—complications may occur

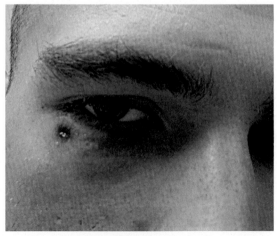

Fig. 13.17 A 37-year-old man who suffered BB injury to the right lower eyelid. The entry site is visible.

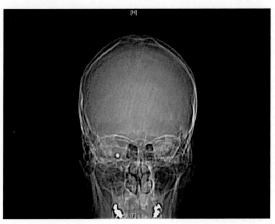

Fig. 13.18 Plain film x-ray showing BB lodged in the right orbit.

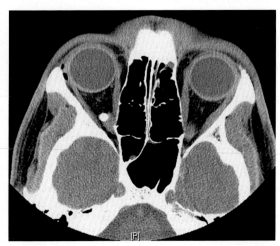

Fig. 13.19 Axial CT scan showing the BB in the posterior portion of the orbit. Ocular functions were normal.

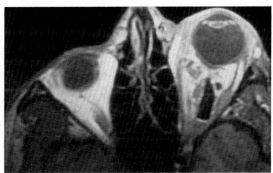

Fig. 13.20 A T_1-weighted MRI showing a hypointense mass in the orbit that represented a piece of retained wood. The patient was admitted for treatment of orbital cellulitis, and the wood was surgically removed.

Orbital Hemorrhage

Key Facts

- Most commonly occurs from accidental trauma
  - Less common after surgery
  - Rarely spontaneous
- Main concern is increased orbital pressure that may lead to vision loss via optic nerve compression and/or elevated IOP
- If vision is threatened, orbital pressure must be normalized, usually by performing a lateral canthotomy and cantholysis
- Most hemorrhages resolve without any treatment
- If possible, any medication affecting coagulation should be discontinued before elective orbital or eyelid surgery
- **Certain conditions more susceptible to spontaneous hemorrhage, such as:**
  - varix • lymphangioma • arteriovenous malformation
- May present associated with primary malignancy
- An uncommon complication of retrobulbar blocks

Clinical Findings

- Sudden onset of orbital pressure or pain
- Swelling of eyelids
  - Chemosis and proptosis can occur if hemorrhage is severe
- **Evaluate:**
  - visual acuity • IOP • proptosis • motility • central retinal artery blood flow

Ancillary Testing

- CT can be helpful to diagnose cause and determine location and extent of hemorrhage

Differential Diagnosis

- Few lesions will be confused with orbital hemorrhage if a history of trauma or surgery precedes
- Spontaneous hemorrhage can be caused by a number of orbital conditions, including orbital malignancy or vascular lesions such as lymphangioma or varix
  - Many rare causes of spontaneous hemorrhage (e.g. scurvy, pregnancy, scuba diving) have been reported

Treatment

- If vision is unaffected, IOP not significantly elevated, and central retinal artery open, observe
- **If optic nerve function is compromised:**
  - open any surgical wound, remove hematoma, obtain hemostasis, consider draining wound
  - lateral canthotomy or cantholysis for trauma
  - if visual function is not restored, consider orbital decompression
- Prevent postoperative hemorrhage by discontinuing anticoagulants before elective orbital or eyelid surgery
  - Use meticulous intraoperative hemostasis

Prognosis

- Most hemorrhages resolve without treatment and do not damage vision
- Surgery to normalize orbital pressure can restore blood flow to optic nerve
  - However, if treatment is delayed visual recovery may not be complete

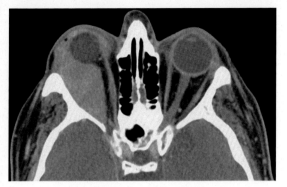

Fig. 13.21 Axial CT showing a large mass in the lateral orbit of a 42-year-old man. This hemorrhage was secondary to recurrent malignant melanoma.

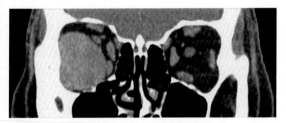

Fig. 13.22 Coronal CT showing the expansile nature of the orbital hemorrhage. Note the medial displacement of the recti muscles and optic nerve.

Section

14

Disorders of the Orbit: Anophthalmic Socket

Enucleation, Evisceration, and Exenteration

Key Facts
- Enucleation is the removal of the entire globe, including cornea, sclera, and a portion of the optic nerve • Evisceration is the removal of the cornea and contents of the globe, leaving the sclera and optic nerve in place • Exenteration is the removal of most of the orbital contents

Surgical Indications
- **Enucleation:**
  - treatment of choice for intraocular tumors or when a pathologic specimen is indicated • effective for blind, painful eyes, intraocular infection, and irreparably traumatized eyes • longer and more complicated procedure than evisceration
- **Evisceration:**
  - contraindicated for intraocular tumors and severe phthisis • considered by some to be treatment of choice for blind eyes with severe intraocular infection • effective for blind painful eyes • faster, less complicated surgery than enucleation • can be done with a retrobulbar block • may provide less protection against sympathetic ophthalmia than enucleation, but unproven • may provide better motility
- **Exenteration:**
  - indicated for infiltrative malignancies of orbit • can be primary orbital malignancies (e.g. adenoid cystic carcinoma of lacrimal gland) or secondary malignancies (e.g. orbital extension of cutaneous basal or squamous cell cancers)

Sympathetic Ophthalmia

- Rare, bilateral, granulomatous panuveitis of unknown cause after penetrating ocular trauma or surgery • Non-injured eye "sympathizes" with the injured eye • Enucleation within 10 days of injury thought to prevent sympathetic ophthalmia • Debate continues as to prophylactic effectiveness of evisceration
- Treated with oral steroids
  - Management is difficult in many cases

Preoperative Considerations

- **Alternatives to enucleation or evisceration:**
  - steroid, cycloplegic, or antiglaucoma drops for pain control • custom scleral shell for cosmesis over blind, disfigured, but pain-free eye • retrobulbar alcohol injection is painful, rarely indicated or effective
- **Alternatives to exenteration:**
  - exenteration indicated only if surgery is likely to provide cure • radiation and/or chemotherapy for palliation

Surgical Technique

- **Enucleation:**
  - 360° limbal peritomy • identify, detach, and tag the recti muscles (double-armed 5-0 Vicryl [polyglactin] suture) • cut the oblique muscles from globe • clamp optic nerve with a large hemostat • transect optic nerve anterior to clamp • cauterize optic nerve stump and release clamp • attach recti muscles to implant • close Tenon's capsule and conjunctiva with 5-0 and 7-0 Vicyl suture • place conformer and pressure patch
- **Evisceration:**
  - 360° limbal peritomy • remove cornea and adjacent 2–3 mm of sclera • remove intraocular contents with evisceration spoon • some surgeons clean sclera with absolute alcohol to remove pigment • radial scleral relaxing incisions allow for implant placement • place implant (typically polymethylmethacrylate [PMMA] implant 16–22 mm, typically 20 mm) • some surgeons open posterior sclera to allow larger implant to extend into intraconal space • close scleral over implant with 5-0 Mersilene suture • close Tenon's capsule and conjunctiva with 5-0 Vicryl suture • place conformer and pressure patch

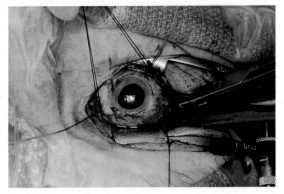

Fig. 14.1 Transecting the optic nerve anterior to the hemostat.

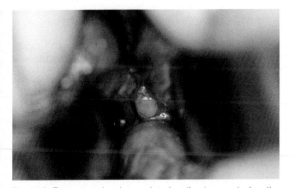

Fig. 14.2 Retractors in place, showing the transected optic nerve stump.

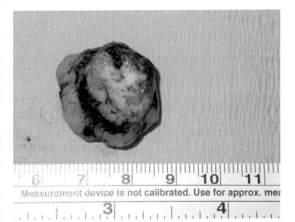

Fig. 14.3 Dermis fat graft before implantation.

Implant Options

- **Choice of implant depends on:**
  - patient's age and health • socket condition • potential peg placement • surgery performed
- Most implants now placed without a separate covering
  - Materials used to wrap implant include donor or processed sclera, fascia, or pericardium; autologous sclera or fascia; and Vicryl (polyglactin) mesh
- Implant materials
  Porous, integrated implants:
  - made of polyethylene (Medpor) or hydroxyapatite (Bio-Eye) • expensive when compared with PMMA spheres • polyethylene implants now made with preplaced holes for muscle attachment with a smooth anterior surface allowing for placement without wrapping • hydroxyapatite implants historically have required wrapping material to allow for muscle attachment, now made with synthetic coating material • become vascularized • some surgeons chose to "peg" hydroxyapatite implants for better motility • polyethylene implants can have a screw placed on anterior surface • a magnetic attachment of the Medpor implant to the prosthesis has recently become available
  Solid, non-integrated, PMMA spheres:
  - an alternative economical choice if peg placement is not planned • good choice for evisceration • wrapping required for enucleation unless implant placed posterior to Tenon's capsule • higher risk of extrusion
  Dermis fat graft:
  - 20-mm circular piece of dermis with underlying adipose tissue (harvested from buttock or belly) • best for sockets with excessive scarring or conjunctival tissue loss, infection, previous extrusion, or poor vascularity • muscles can be attached to graft • provides less motility

Surgical Complications of Enucleation or Evisceration

- Exposure, extrusion, infection, ectropion, ptosis, superior sulcus defect, giant papillary conjunctivitis (see *Care and complications of the anophthalmic socket*)

Surgical Technique for Exenteration

- Skin incisions made to orbital rim, preserving orbital septum and exposing entire orbital rim • Periosteum is cut and periorbita elevated off orbital walls • A clamp is placed, enclosing the orbital tissues
- Orbital tissues are cut with curved scissors and delivered
  - The apical tissues are cauterized
- Socket can be grafted with meshed split-thickness skin grafts or allowed to granulate in place
- In cases in which apical tissues are involved but there is no anterior involvement, the eyelid skin can be preserved
  - In rare cases, the eyelids and conjunctival fornices can be saved • The socket is usually filled with a free flap
- An oculofacial prosthesis can be fashioned
  - Bone-anchored implants (osseointegration) can be placed • Magnetic attachments align and retain the prosthesis against the socket • Alternatively, a black patch can be used to cover the defect

Prognosis

- Excellent cosmesis and comfort typical after enucleation or evisceration along with custom ocular prosthesis
  - Patients undergoing exenteration may wear a black patch or an oculofacial prosthesis

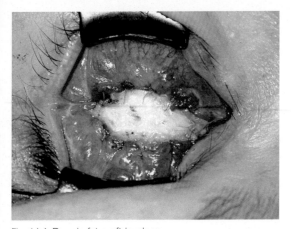

Fig. 14.4 Dermis fat graft in place.

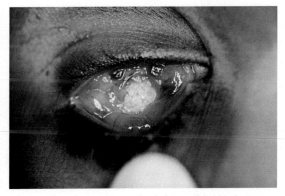

Fig. 14.5 Exposed porous polyethylene orbital implant.

Care and Complications of the Anophthalmic Socket

Key Facts

- Fit prosthesis 6–8 weeks postoperatively
  - Keep conformer in place until prosthesis
- Custom prosthesis with modified impression fitting technique
- Patient should minimize handling of prosthesis but check socket once every month or two
- Lack of lubrication is most common cause of irritation
- Prosthesis should be cleaned annually by an ocularist
- Socket should be inspected annually by an ophthalmologist
- Prosthesis should be replaced every 7–10 years routinely—sooner if fitting problems develop

Clinical Findings

- Common anophthalmic problems
  Superior sulcus syndrome (Fig. 14.6):
  - high sulcus contributing to ptotic-appearing upper eyelid
  - caused by laxity of lower and inadequate orbital volume
  - lax lower eyelid allows prosthesis to drop
  - volume loss may be due to fat atrophy, absence, or undersized implant
  Giant papillary conjunctivitis:
  - mucoid discharge
  - giant papillae on tarsal conjunctiva (Fig. 14.7)
  - immunologic reaction, probably against the plastic
  Entropion:
  - inversion of eyelashes usually due to posterior lamellar shrinkage caused a poor-fitting eye (Fig. 14.8)
  - an extreme version of conjunctival shrinkage is known as socket contraction—patients lose the fornices and cannot wear a prosthesis, and correction is difficult
  Implant exposure:
  - conjunctival and Tenon's capsule defect (Fig. 14.9)
  - a large area of exposure predisposes patient to infection and may allow implant to extrude
  - in general, a porous Implant that becomes exposed will not extrude because connective tissue growing into the implant holds it in the socket
  Ptosis:
  - caused by normal involutional causes or as a result of eyelid trauma at the same time as any ocular injury
  - loss of volume (see above) can contribute to ptotic appearance (see pseudoptosis section)

Ancillary Testing

- None

Differential Diagnosis

- Recurrent tumor should be ruled out as cause of discharge or poorly fitting eye
- Routine problems such as conjunctivitis or dacryocystitis can occur in anophthalmic socket

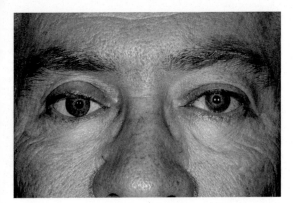

Fig. 14.6 Superior sulcus syndrome: note sunken appearance to eye, ptotic eyelid, and globe ptosis.

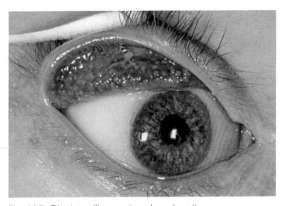

Fig. 14.7 Giant papillae on tarsal conjunctiva.

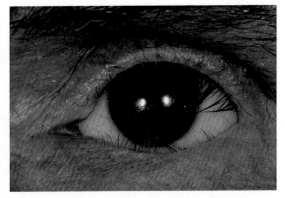

Fig. 14.8 Implant exposure: conjunctival and Tenon's capsule defect around old style tantalum mesh implant.

Treatment

- **Discharging socket:**
  - if no problem is identified, try lubrication using artificial tears, mineral oral, or vitamin E oil
- **Superior sulcus syndrome:**
  - if no implant is present, place an 18- or 20-mm implant
  - if lower eyelid laxity is present, tighten lower lid using a lateral tarsal strip
  - if volume is still inadequate, add a subperiosteal implant (Fig. 14.9)—do not make a larger prosthesis
- **Giant papillary conjunctivitis:**
  - polish eye if it is <7 years old
  - new prosthesis if polishing does not work or prosthesis is old
  - lubricate (for refractory cases, use topical steroid drops one to four times daily)
- **Entropion:**
  - lid margin–everting procedures such as the tarsal fracture (see *Trichiasis: marginal entropion and other causes*)
  - mucous membrane grafting for severe cases
- **Implant exposure:**
  - small exposures may be observed for a short period; if no healing, close defect with undermining or close over a scleral patch
  - larger exposures or extrusions can be treated by placing a smaller implant if adequate conjunctiva is present
  - if conjunctival closure compromises the depth of the fornices, a dermis fat graft should be placed, which will restore volume and conjunctiva
- **Ptosis:**
  - minor amounts of ptosis can be corrected by modifying prosthesis to lift eyelid slightly
  - for more severe ptosis, levator aponeurosis advancement or frontalis sling

Prognosis

- Most patients can successfully wear an ocular prosthesis comfortably and inconspicuously
  - Minimal or no discharge is the norm

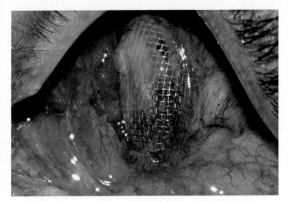

Fig. 14.9 Entropion of eyelids due to a poorly fitting prosthesis.

Index

Index

N

O

Orbital trauma, 242–257
    computerized tomography, 154, 155
Orbital varix, 238–239, 256

Pain
    adenoid cystic carcinoma of lacrimal
        gland, 222, 223
    blowout orbital fracture, 244
    idiopathic orbital inflammation, 178
    orbital bacterial cellulitis, 162
    orbital hemorrhage, 256
    orbital metastases, 228, 229
    orbital varix, 238
Paralytic ectropion, 84–87
Paralytic entropion, 97
Parinaud syndrome, 116
Pediatric tumors, 224
    metastatic orbital, 224–227
Plain film X-ray, intraorbital foreign body,
    254, 255
Plexiform neurofibroma, 204
Posterior lamellar scarring, 96
Preseptal cellulitis, 160–161
Proptosis
    adenoid cystic carcinoma of lacrimal
        gland, 222, 223
    benign mixed tumor of lacrimal gland,
        220, 221
    cavernous hemangioma, 196
    dermoid cyst, 190
    lymphangioma, 198
    neurofibroma, 204, 205
    optic nerve glioma, 200, 201
    orbital arteriovenous fistula, 236
    orbital bacterial cellulitis, 162
    orbital hemorrhage, 256
    orbital metastases
        adult, 228, 229, 230, 232
        pediatric, 224, 226
    orbital varix, 238
    rhabdomyosarcoma, 212, 213, 215
    sarcoidosis, 180
    sphenoid wing meningioma, 208
    thyroid orbitopathy, 174, 175, 176
Prostate cancer, orbital/choroidal
    metastases, 228, 230, 232, 233
Pseudoptosis, 114–115
Ptosis
    acquired involutional, 102–105
    anophthalmic socket, 264, 266
    blepharophimosis syndrome, 10
    brow, 68–69
    chalazion, 28
    congenital myogenic, 2–5

floppy eyelid syndrome, 70
hordeolum, 28
Horner syndrome, 108, 109
involutional ectropion, 80
myasthenia gravis, 110, 111, 112, 113
neurofibroma, 204, 205
rhabdomyosarcoma, 215
sarcoidosis, 180
third nerve palsy, 106–107
Punch biopsy, 47
    cutaneous melanoma, 56
    lentigo maligna, 42
Punctate keratopathy
    epiblepharon, 6
    floppy eyelid syndrome, 70
    involutional entropion, 92
Punctoplasty, canaliculitis curettage, 146,
    147

Radiation therapy complications, 214
Reactive lymphoid hyperplasia, 216
Reflex spasm, 120, 124
Retinal vasculitis
    sarcoidosis, 180
    Wegener granulomatosis, 184
Rhabdomyosarcoma, 212–215
    histologic subtypes, 214
    pediatric orbital metastases, 224

Saddle nose deformity, Wegener
    granulomatosis, 184, 186
Salmon patch, conjunctival lymphoma, 217
Sarcoidosis, 154, 180–183
Scleritis
    idiopathic orbital inflammation, 178
    Wegener granulomatosis, 184
Sebaceous adenocarcinoma (sebaceous cell
    carcinoma), 52–55
Seborrheic blepharitis, 22, 23, 25
Seborrheic dermatitis, 22
Seborrheic keratosis, 30–31
Shave biopsy, 47
    seborrheic keratosis, 30
Silent sinus syndrome, 246
Sinus disease, 154
Sinusitis
    orbital bacterial cellulitis, 162, 164, 165
    preseptal cellulitis, 160
Sixth nerve palsy, orbital arteriovenous
    fistula, 236
Snap-back test, 76
Sphenoid wing meningioma, 156, 208–211

Printed in the United States
By Bookmasters